Vinca Twins: Cell Division & Cancer Control

Jacob

Copyright © 2024 by Jacob

INDEX.

<u>CHAPTER 1.</u>

THE   CHOICE   OF   A SYSTEM.

CHAPTER 1.

The Choice of a System.

Vincristine and vinblastine, two closely related
alkaloids are extracted from the Madagaskar Periwinkle,
Vinca rosea Linn. They have been shown to be effective
oncolytic agents and cause arrest of mitosis at the
metaphase stage, similar to that of colchicine and
colcimid.

Clinically, vincristine has been found to produce
a complete remission in patients with acute leukaemia.
Tumour regression in patients with Hodgkin's disease,
lymphosarcoma and certain childhood solid tumours have
also been reported (Palmer, 1960; Armstrong, et al, 1961.)

Clinical studies with vincristine and vinblastine
have been carried out in the Radiotherapy Department
of the Groote Schuur Hospital. For example, with the
aid of these alkaloids, the potential doubling times
of human squamous carcinomas have been determined,
(Sealy, and Greenstein, 1971).

Vincristine was found to posess antitumour, antimitotic, stathmokinetic and toxic properties. The
mechanism of the stathmokinetic property remains obscure.
Although the morphological effects are indistinguishable
from that produced by colchicine, the overall biological
effects of colchicine are dissimilar to those of the
alkaloids.

Research programmes in the Department of Bio-
Engineering and Medical Physics are being conducted
on various biological systems, to determine the mode
of action of the alkaloids. These systems are: the
cheek pouch of the Syrian hamster, Hela and Elhrich-
ascites cells in culture, and the root meristem of
Vicia faba.

The reason for choosing Vicia faba as a tool
for the study of radiomimetic properties of drugs,
is that the cell parameters of the bean root are known
with great accuracy. In the past, seedlings of Vicia
faba have been used to investigate biological effects
of ionizing radiation. As early as 1913, Mottram,
then Director of Research at the Mount Vernon Hospital,
reported effects of radiation on Vicia seedlings.

Just before the Second World War, Read began a
detailed investigation of the gross effects shown by
roots after irradiation, namely reduction or cessation
of growth. (Read, 1952) .

Since then the root meristem of Vicia faba has
been used by a widening circle of workers, and it is
probable that today more is known about its response to
radiation than about any other biological system.
Pioneering work on Vicia includes investigations by
Kumoro (1922-31), Jüngling (1923-32), and Ingber (1931-32).

A great deal of work has been done by botanists on
the cell population kinetics of the root meristem of
Vicia faba. Radiation has often been a tool for their

studies. The work of Clowes (1959) on the quiescent centre is notable in this respect. Hall, Lajtha and Oliver (1962) have, on the other hand, used the population kinetics of the root and deduced the dose response relations with respect to the reproductive integrity of the meristematic cells.

As important consideration in choosing _Vicia_ as a system to work on is the cost involved. Plant systems have the advantage of cheapness of materials, and the ability to handle large enough numbers to reduce experimental errors to a reasonable level. Also, plant systems are favourable above animal systems because of the suffering which animals experience. Irradiation of root systems is also much simpler than the procedures taken to irradiate animals.

Vicia has an added advantage above most other systems; the effect of x-rays and radiomimetic drugs can be assessed conveniently by the growth reduction of the primary root. Also, the meristem of _Vicia_ contains a small number of large chromosomes, and simple cytological analysis can easily be made. Many studies have been made of the histology and cytology of the root tip, so that the ability of radiation to produce mitotic delay/chromosome and aberration have been investigated in detail.

Read (1952) has demonstrated the influence of oxygen on the response of living cells to ionizing radiation. Read and Gray, (1959) have shown that close parallels

exist between the responses of the bean root and those
of other organisms and human tissue. Vincristine has
been found to be a radiomimetic drug, it is thus
believed that an extrapolation of results with
vincristine on _Vicia faba_ to the human situation is
possible.

THE QUANTITATIVE BASIS OF RADIOBIOLOGY

CHAPTER 2

"THE QUANTITATIVE BASIS OF RADIOBIOLOGY"

Before discussing the morphology of _Vicia faba_ and its root, it is necessary to examine some of the radiobiological background.

Dose Response Curves.

The effect of radiation on biological functions is usually studied by determining the variation in that function with increase in dose, yielding what is known as a dose-response curve.

In 1956 Puck and Marcus described a technique of colony culture _in vitro_ for mammalian cells, which permitted the determination of the x-ray dose-response curve of these cells with respect to their reproductive integrity. Later Hewitt and Wilson (1959) described a technique for determination of such a dose response curve for mouse leukaemia cells _in vivo_. Since then both these methods have been applied by other workers (e.g. Elkind and Sutton, 1959; Barensen _et al_, 1960; Berry and Andrews, 1963; Berry, 1969).

A typical dose-response curve showing the surviving fraction of hamster fibroblast cells plotted against dose in rads is shown in Fig. 2.1. The mathematical derivation and meaning of the symbols used will be discussed later in this chapter.

.5.

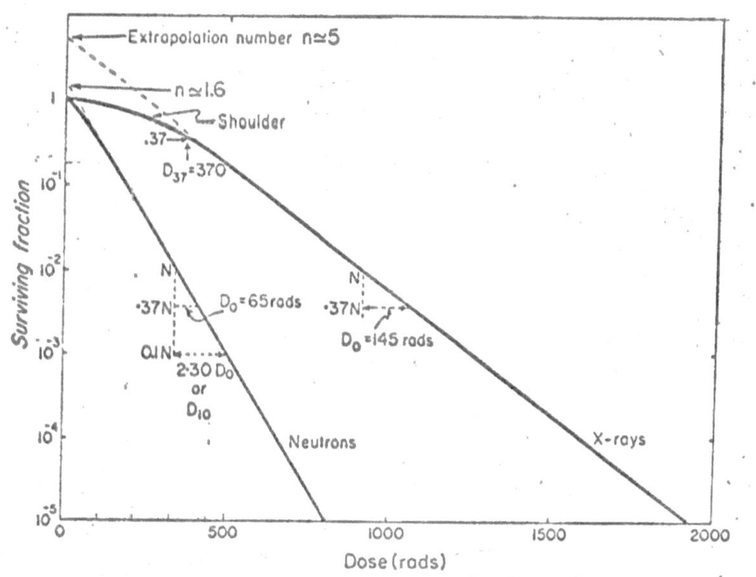

Fig. 2.1 A typical dose – response curve showing the surviving fraction of hamster fibroblast cells plotted against dose in rads. (Whitmore, 1964).

The Shape of Survival Curves.

To explain the shape of survival curves, it is convenient to speak of the region in which ionization has to be produced to obtain mutation, killing or other effect studies as the target. The passage of the ionizing particle may be spoken of as a hit.

Consider the type of action caused by a single hit: it is evident that the number of hits is simply proportional to the dose of radiation given. If the dose given is such that only a small proportion of the targets are hit, no distinction need be made between the total number of hits and the number of targets hit. The number of targets hit is then proportional to the dose, and a straight line is obtained by plotting the yield of the reaction against the dose.

If the dose is larger, so that the number of targets
hit is a considerable proportion of the whole number,
cases will occur of several hits being obtained in a single
target. The number of targets hit will then be less than
the number of hits. Although the total number of hits
increases in strict proportionality to the dose, the
number of targets hit increases more slowly, so that the
yield plotted against the dose gives a curve which is
convex upwards tending asymptotically to 100%.

If one is following, say, the killing of bacteria or
single-celled organisms, the _numbers_ killed by successive
increments of dose is not equal, but each increment of
dose kills the same _proportion_ of the numbers of organisms
which have survived until then. The number of viable
organisms falls off in a geometrical progression, i.e. the
survival curve is sigmoid, as in Fig. 2.1.

<u>The Hit and Target Theories</u>.

Theories, explaining the shape of survival curves,
will be discussed in this and following sections.

The basic idea of the <u>hit theory</u> by Dessauer (1922)
can be stated as follows: the reaction to be studies
(e.g. lethality, loss of reproductive integrity, appearance
of chromosomes aberations), occurs to a particular one out
of a great number of irradiated individuals (e.g. cell
populations) if a determinable number (hit number) of
hits occur in that single individual. Since the region

in which the hit number must occur need not be identical
with the volume of the individual each individual can
have one or more targets ascribed to it.

According to this view, the form of the observed
dose response curve is due to the fact that obsorption
or radiation is not continuous, but a quantized process
which follows a Poisson distribution.

Target theory (Crowther, 1924) concerns itself with
concept of a "hit" or a "hit event", since the most varied
types of chemical processes can be visualised as such
"events" in so far as they transfer energy from radiation
to matter. This concept offers the possibility of
calculating from the dose-response a volume, i.e., the
target, within which the required number of these
absorption events must occur during irradiation with
given probability.

Exponential Inactivation

Suppose a biological sample, which contains N biological
entities (these entities may be enzyme molecules, viruses,
tumour cells, etc.), is given a small dose of radiation dD.
It is required to calculate the number of entities dN which
are inactivated by this dose dD. The number of inactiva-
tions produced should be proportional to the dose and in
proportion to the number of entities present. This state-
ment may be expressed mathematically by

$$dN = -\frac{1}{D_o} N \, dD \qquad \ldots\ldots\ldots 2.1$$

where $\frac{1}{D_o}$ is a constant of proportionality. D_o'
represents a dose, because dN and N have the same
dimensions.

Rearranging, e.g. 2.1 becomes

$$dD = - \frac{dN}{N} \quad D_o \ldots\ldots\ldots\ldots 2.2$$

If dN is made equal to N, then D_o is the dose that
would be required to inactivate all the entities if
they continued to be inactivated at the initial rate
of inactivation. The quantity D_o is called the mean
lethal dose and is the dose that is required on the
average to place one inactivating event ("hit") in
each of the biological entities.

Equations 2.1 and 2.2 only apply to very small
increments in dose dD.. They may be integrated to give

$$N = N_o e^{- D/D_o} \quad \ldots\ldots\ldots\ldots 2.3$$

where N is the number of unaffected biological entities
present, after dose D, and N_o is the initial number
present.

If $D = D_o$, e.g. 2.3 becomes

$$N = N_o e^{- 1} \quad \text{or} \quad N = 0.37 \, N_o$$

Thus, the mean lethal dose is the dose required
to reduce the population of entities to 37 per cent
of its initial value, and thus destroy 63 per cent of
the population.

Typical survival curves for a line of hamster cells
exposed to x-rays and neutrons are given in Fig. 2.1.
From equation 2.3, a straight line is expected if N/N_o

(the surviving fraction) is plotted against dose
on semilogarithmic paper. This is nearly the case
for neutrons, but low x-ray doses show a pronounced
"shoulder". The curves become straight at large
doses, so that equation 2.3 applies to large doses.

D_o is obtained from the straight portion and
is the dose required to reduce the number of
surviving cells from any value N to 0.37N as
indicated in Fig. 2.1.

Multi-Target Survival Curves.

It can be shown (e.g. Zirkle, 1952; Fowler, 1964)
that the general form of the survival curve for
identical individuals having m targets, each requiring
a minimum of n hits before the individual is inactivated,
is given by:

$$S = 1 - (1-B)^m \quad \ldots\ldots\ldots\ldots (2.4)$$

$$\text{where} \quad B = e^{-x}\left(1 + X + \frac{X^2}{2!} + \ldots \frac{X^{(n-1)}}{(n-1)!}\right) \ldots\ldots (2.5)$$

$$\text{and} \quad X = D/D_o$$

S is the surviving fraction after dose D (rads)
and D_o is the dose (in rads) to give an average of one
"hit" in each formal target volume.

The multi-target model is derived by assuming
that only one hit is required in each of m targets,
i.e. n = 1 and therefore B = exp $(-D/D_o)$

The resulting survival curve is of the form:

$$S = 1 - \left\{1 - \exp(D/D_o)\right\}^m \quad \ldots\ldots\ldots\ldots 2.6$$

Expansion of equation 2.6 indicates that for large doses, the higher terms are negligible and under these conditions the relationship approximates to:

$$S = m \exp\left(-D/D_o\right)$$

so that $\ln S = \ln m - D/D_o$

Thus, if the log of the surviving fraction is plotted against dose on a linear scale, after an initial shoulder, a straight-line graph is obtained with a slope determined by $- D/D_o$ and extrapolating back to intercept the ordinate scale at m. This form has been called a Type C survival curve by Gunter and Kohn (1956).   (Oliver & Shepstone, 1964)

CHAPTER 3.

THE MORPHOLOGY OF THE ROOT

VICIA FABA

The Morphology of the Root of <u>Vicia faba</u>.

The species <u>Vicia faba</u> belongs to the genus of <u>Viciaceae</u>, of the <u>Leguminosae</u> family. General features of the fruit and seed of species belonging to this family are: the pistil is monocarpellary. The ovary is one-celled, and bears several ovules, arranged in one or two rows along the ventral suture. The fruit is termed a legume and is strictly so when it is dry along the dorsal suture. The embryo is large, the cotelydons are flat or plano-convex, and the radicle is superior and incurved.

<u>The Development of the Seed.</u>

The seed itself is a very complex structure, composed of a plant embryo, a seed coat, and a supply of stored food.

The mature embryo of <u>Vicia faba</u> consists of an axis bearing two cotelydons, or seed leaves. At the summit of the axis, above the cotyledonary node, is the plumule. This is the apex of the embryonic shoot, and is composed of the apical meristem together with embryonic leaves.

At germination, the plumule gives rise to that portion of the shoot above the cotelydons. The tapering end of the embryo, called the radicle, develops into the primary root when the seed germinates.

<u>The Structure of the Root Tip</u>.

In the root tip of <u>Vicia faba</u> there are three
tiers of initials (permanently meristematic cells)
in the initial zone. One gives rise to the stele or
central cylinder, the second to the cortex and the
third to the root cap. The epidermis differentiates
from the outermost layer of the cortex and arises from
the same initials.

The stele is separated from the root cap by a
single layer of cells at the pole. This layer is part
of the cortex-epidermis complex and its cells form the
distal surface of the quiescent centre (see next section).
The elongating zone extends to about 4 mm from the tip of
the root. Fig. 3.1. represents a section through the
primary root of <u>Vicia</u>, showing the position of the
quiescent centre in relation to other parts of the root.
Fig. 3.2. represents a median section of the normal root
apex according to Clowes (1963) and Hall (1962). The
shaded area represents the quiescent centre.

Fig. 3.3. represents a section through the primary
root. Starting from the tip upwards, it may be divided
approximately in the following sections:

1. The root cap, which occupies the first $\frac{1}{3}$ mm
of the root tip, the cells of which are relatively
inert. As the root pushes forward between the
soil particles by growth in the zone of
elongation, the root tip is protected from
mechanical injury by the root cap. The cells

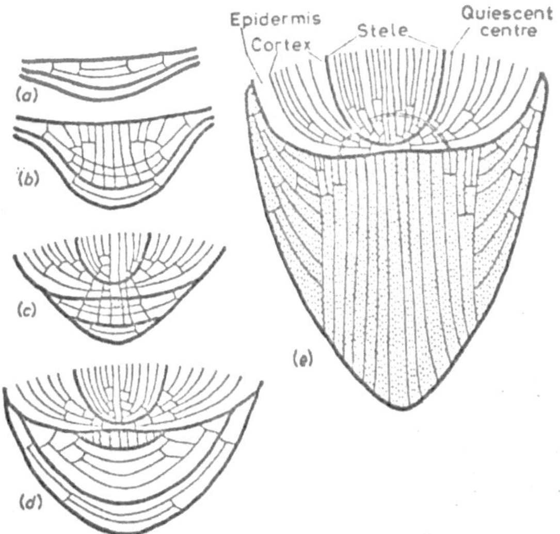

Fig. 3.1 . A section through the primary root of <u>Zea</u>
<u>mays</u>, showing the position of the quiescent centre
in relation to other parts of the root.   (Clowes, 1959).

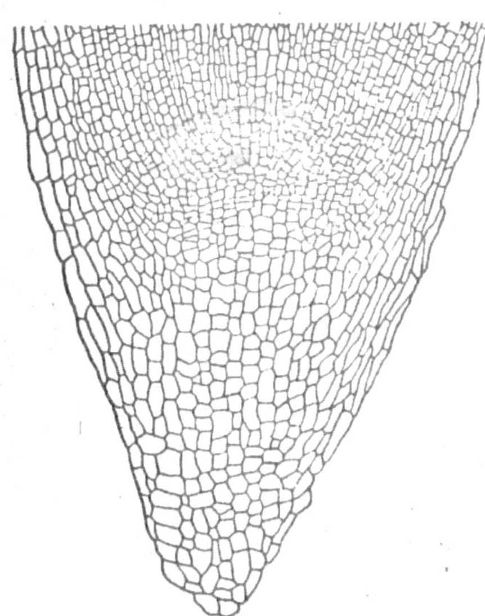

Fig. 3.2. Median section of the root apex of <u>Vicia faba</u>
showing the position of the quiescent centre. (Clowes,1962

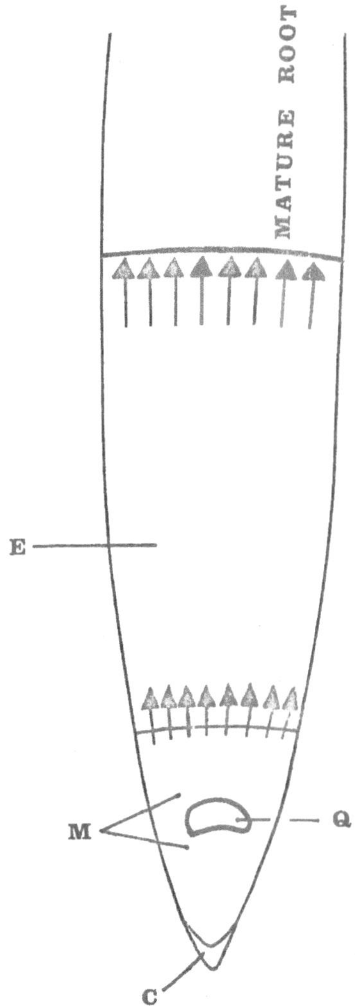

Fig. 3.3. A section through the primary root of _Vicia faba_.
M = meristematic zone.   C = cap.
E = èlongating zone.
Q = quiescent centre. (Clowes, 1959).

15.

of the root cap are renewed from within in
various ways, depending on the species.

2. The meristem occupies the next 3 mm of the root.
   The cells of this zone, like those in the apex of
   the stem, are small, thin-walled and filled with
   protoplasm. Vacuoles are small and numerous.
   Cell division of the apical meristematic cells
   adds little to the length of the root. For a
   normal, unirradiated root, the dividing cells
   have an intermitotic interval of 24 hours at 25°C.

3. Some of the daughter cells from division in the
   meristematic zone become part of the region
   directly behind it, the zone of elongation. Cell
   division may proceed for a time in the latter zone
   but cell enlargement, chiefly by elongation,
   predominates. The elongation of cells causes an
   increase in the length of the root.

4. The remainder of the root is build up of mature
   cells which are fully elongated. Maturation
   involves the development of undifferentiated,
   nonspecialised cells into specialised cells that
   play various roles in the activities of the root.

<u>The Concept of Initial Cells</u>.

Ever since a single 'apical cell' was discovered
in the root meristem of ferns, attempts have been
made to interpret the cell pattern in seed plants
such as <u>Vicia faba</u> as if there were also a single
totipotent cell.

Clowes (1959) suggested that the 'initials' were
situated around the surface of the 'quiescent centre' -
the cells of which divide very infrequently under normal
circumstances.

These studies were a direct result of research
based on the so-called "Körper-Kappe" theory, which
describes the planes of cell division by an analysis
of the pattern of cells (Clowes, 1968). This theory is
an improvement on the histogen theory of Hanstein (1868),
which divided the meristem into three regions, according
to whether they produce stele, cortex or epidermis.
The difficulty of the latter theory is that it cannot
explain how the histogens are maintained and it merely
divides the meristem into regions based on the assumed
differentiation of their cells. Recent investigations
have shown that a combination of the Körper-Kappe theory
with a modified histogen theory adequately explains the
pattern of cells in root meristems. Cells from various
geometrical parts of the root would thus constitute the
initials of the several anatomical regions of the root
e.g. the meristematic cells above the quiescent centre
initiate the stele and cortex, while those below initiate
the root cap.(Guttenberg, 1955; Popham, 1955; Clowes, 1954).

The Quiescent Centre.

From a geometrical analysis of the pattern of
division in apical meristems, Clowes (1954) postulated
the existence in root apices of _Zea_ of a quiescent centre -
a region in which the cells divide rarely, if at all, in
the normal growth of the root.

Clowes reasoned that the pattern of cells in the
root apex of _Zea mays_ is such that unambiguous conclusions
can be drawn about the planes of division, and the relative
rate of division. The central rows in the caps do not
divide longitudinally and therefore do not grow transversely.
This means that the cells at the pole of the cortex-
epidermis complex also do not divide longitudinally, and
it is known that they do not divide transversely, because
on the axis, there is only one layer of cells between the
clearly defined boundaries of the stele and cap. Thus
Clowes was able to conclude that the cells at the pole
of the stele and cortex-epidermis complex do not divide
at all.

The constituent cells of the quiescent centre are
carried forward passively by the growth of the surrounding
meristem and contribute few cells to the root. They are
quiescent only because of their position within the apex,
and not because of any inherent disability. The pattern
of growth in a root meristem can change both spontaneously
and when stimulated, and when this happens, cells in the
quiescent centre can become meristematic (Clowes, 1962).

Whilst the geometrical approach does not give
unambiguous results when applied to root apices of the
other species of plants with poorly defined tissue
boundaries, other methods show that there is a quiescent
centre in all roots except for those with a single apical
cell. (Clowes, 1962, 1959).

The existence of the quiescent centre was proved
by feeding _Vicia faba_ roots with radioactive D N A
precursors. In autoradiographs of prepared root sections,
the quiescent centre was clearly demarcated from the
remainder of the meristem because the labelled D N A
precursors were incorporated at a much slower rate,
indicating infrequent cell division. This method has
also been used to measure rates of mitosis (Clowes, 1968).

In _Vicia faba_, the quiescent centre cells are grouped
together in a hemispherically shaped volume. About 1000
out of 250000 actively dividing cells occupy the quiescent
centre. _Zea mays_ has roughly 600 cells compared to 125000
actively dividing cells in the quiescent centre.

The table below shows the average duration of the
mitotic cycle (in hours) in three regions of root meristems
for _Zea mays_ and _Vicia faba_.

	Quiescent Centre	Cap Initials	Stele
Zea mays	174	12	28
Vicia faba	292	44	37

(Clowes, 1968)

Sinapsis, Pistia and Eichhornia roots showed a
sharply delineated boundary between the quiescent
centre and the contiguous cap initials. The proximal
boundary is not always as clear. At present one can
only speculate about what it is that maintains such
a big difference in rates of cell division in contiguous
cells, but with differences of the order of 15-fold
one would expect to find also other differences in the
cells of the regions of the meristem. The quiescent
centre must have lower rates of synthesis than the rest
of the meristem. This has been proved true for D N A
and protein (Clowes, 1959), and the cells of the quiescent
centre are known to have less D N A and protein and, on
the average, less D N A than other parts of the apex
(Jensen, 1958). They have smaller nuclei, smaller
nucleoli, smaller Golgi bodies, fewer mitochondria per
cell, and less endoplasmic reticulum. All these features
change abruptly in passing from the quiescent centre to the
cap initials, and all of them can be related to the
difference in rate of mitosis (Clowes, 1963).

Behaviour of the Quiescent Centre after Irradiation.

Generally, after irradiation, the growth of a root
slows down, reaches a minimum after a few days, and then
recovers if the dose is not too high. In earlier
explanations of how the changes in rates of root growth
occurred, it was assumed that all the cells of the
meristem were equally meristematic. To investigate

the behaviour of meristems after irradiation by
autoradiographic methods, roots were fed with precursors
of D N A at various time intervals after irradiation
(Clowes, 1959). From this work it became clear that
the quiescent centre behaved differently from the rest
of the meristem. D N A synthesis stopped in many of
the normally meristematic cells and started in the
previously quiescent cells. There was thus a reversal
in the roles of the two parts of the apex. This
observation has been further investigated by measuring
the rates of mitosis in the same way as in the normal
meristems. The cells in the quiescent centre therefore
form a 'reservoir' of cells which are less vulnerable
because of their quiescence, but are able to restart
D N A synthesis and division when the normally meristematic
cells stop (Clowes, 1959).

The results are summarized in the following table
for <u>Vicia faba</u> subjected to acute irradiation. (Clowes, 1963).

Average Duration of the Mitotic Cycle (in hours) After Acute X-Irradiation.				
Dose (rads)	Days After Irradiation	Quiescent Centre	Cap Initials	Stele
0	–	292	44	37
360	3	65	95	95
360	7	38	55	55
360	10	46	51	58
360	14	162	74	41

(Clowes, 1963).

Population Kinetics in the Root Meristem of <u>Vicia faba</u>

It has been shown that, after three days of
irradiation of Vicia faba roots, the mitotic cycle is
the same as unirradiated roots (Hornsey, 1956).
Consequently, the reduction in growth-rate which is
observed at times later than three days after irradiation,
does not result from a lengthening of the mitotic cycle.
Further, root growth is unaffected by irradiation of the
elongating zone itself, even to a very high dose, provided
the meristem is shielded (Gray and Boag, unpublished;
Cit. Read, 1959). Consequently, the pattern of differentiation
must be determined within the meristem, and is not influenced
by the existing differentiated tissue. This conclusion is
supported by the work of Bünning (1952), Torrey (1955, 1957)
and Ball (1948, 1951), and is discussed in detail by Clowes
(1959).

The fundamental effect of radiation is the loss of
reproductive integrity by a proportion of cells in the cell
population. Hence the sterilizing of meristematic cells
must ultimately account for the reduction in growth (Lea, 1946)
It is therefore logical to conclude that the intermediate
mechanism is the reduction in the number of cells that have
differentiated and are presenting themselves for differentiatio

<u>Theoretical Patterns</u>.

Four different theoretical models of the meristem,
which could explain the normal growth of the root to a
fair degree of satisfaction, have been proposed by different
authors. The first two of these were by Hall, Lajtha and

Oliver (1962), the third by Oliver and Shepstone (1963), and the fourth by Dewey and Howard (1963).

In a control root growing at a constant rate, it is assumed that when a cell differentiates and leaves the meristem to elongate, another meristem divides to maintain the total dividing population at a constant level. In effect, during the course of one cycle, half of the cells in the meristem differentiate, while the other half divide and double in number. The cell population in such a model meristem is thus maintained in a steady state, while providing a continuous and constant supply of cells for elongation.

It is possible to postulate three ways in which the meristematic compartment may be expected to behave after being subjected to a dose of radiation:

(1) The pattern of differentiation within the meristem may be unaltered by the radiation; i.e. in spite of its compartment becoming depopulated as damaged cells die, 50 per cent per cell cycle may still elongate and the remainder divide. If this were true, the growth rate of irradiated roots would fall to a value characteristic of the proportion of cells sterilized, and would remain at this level (see Fig. 3.4.).

This system cannot explain the recovery that is observed in practice.

(2) The second possibility is that the "size" of the meristem may be the all-important factor, and that, once depopulated, production of elongating cells stops until cell proliferation in the meristem restores it to

its original size. Once this has been accomplished,
elongation would re-commence. However, such a system
would result in a temporary cessation of growth, followed
by a sudden recovery to the pre-irradiation level (see
Fig. 3.5). This is not consistent with the observed
facts, since, even after 200 rads, the growth-rate
slows but never becomes zero, and recovery takes place
gradually over a period of several days.

(3) The third possibility is that when the number
of meristematic cells is less than normal as a result of
radiation-induced cell death, then the proportion of
cells which differentiate in a given time interval is
also less than normal. Hall, Lajtha and Oliver (1962)
have considered this postulate in great detail and have
suggested two possible meristematic models, Model A and
Model B. These models will now be discussed, with brief
reference only to the relevant mathematics. A full
mathematical treatment will be given in the appendix.

Model A.

This model assumes that the meristem population is
in exponential growth, this growth being balanced by a
removal mechanism that ensures that the proportion of
cells differentiating is proportional to the fractional
size of the meristem. This would lead to an exponential
distribution of cells within the cell cycle. Following

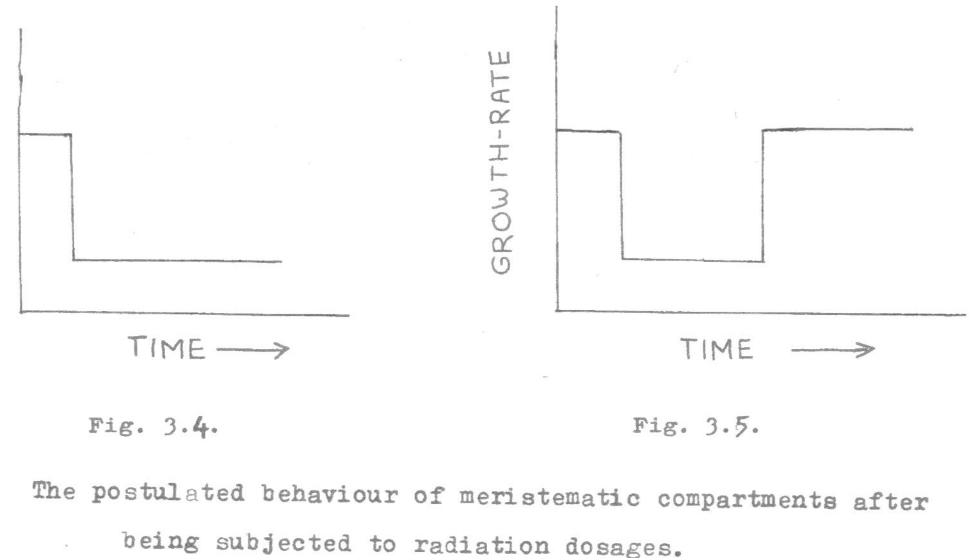

Fig. 3.4.   Fig. 3.5.

The postulated behaviour of meristematic compartments after
being subjected to radiation dosages.

radiation damage, since the intermitotic cycle is
unaltered (Hornsey, 1956), the proportion of cells
dividing in a given time interval is unimpaired and
the meristem is gradually repopulated.

As recovery progresses, the compartment approaches
its normal size, rate of differentiation, and hence root
growth returns to its steady state value. This model
satisfies the observation that the miminum growth rate
decreases with increase in dose, and that the subsequent
recovery is gradual over a period of several days. Also,
the pattern of differentiation is determined within the
apex which is in accord with the conclusions of Clowes (1959).

Hall, Lajtha and Oliver (1962) derive the expression

$$\frac{dD}{dt} = \frac{y\, I_s}{\left\{1 + \left(\frac{Is}{Io} - 1\right) e^{-yt}\right\}^2} \qquad (3.1)$$

for the rate of differentiation, D, at any time in terms
of the number I_o of integer cells in the model meristem
after irradiation. I_s is the number of cells in the
meristem under steady state growth conditions, and the
time constant, y is defined as:

$$y = \frac{\ln 2}{\text{intermitotic period}} \qquad (3.2)$$

In order to simplify the derivation of the above
expression, the authors have assumed that fatally damaged
cells are removed immediately after irradiation. Therefore,
the curve derived from the above equation cannot simply be
matched to experimental growth rate curves to derive the
initial population. Hall and his co-workers avoid this

difficulty by introducing a step-by-step calculation, to trace the attempts by the integer cells in the meristem to repopulate the compartment by division, while assuming that the fraction of cells which differentiate (and are lost from the compartment) depends on the total number of cells present, i.e. integer or sterile, I_t.

The term "integer" when applied to an irradiated cell implies that it has been left reproductively intact and has therefore retained its reproductive integrity.

The basis of calculation is the curve for daily growth rate, "G", as a fraction of that for control roots of equal age. A step-by-step calculation for time intervals of a quarter day has to be made. This type of calculation is inevitably an approximation, but an increase in the number of steps, whilst increasing the accuracy, adds complication. The interval of a quarter day was chosen as a compromise. G is read off from the daily growth curve for each time interval. The rate of differentiation in an irradiated, and therefore depopulated meristem equals $\left(y \dfrac{I_t^2}{I_s} \right)$ and the corresponding quantity for a control root is yI_s. Expressed as a fraction of control roots, the rate of differentiation, and therefore the growth G becomes

$$G = \left(\frac{I_t}{I_s} \right)^2$$

This equation illustrates the basic postulation of the
model, namely, that the rate of differentiation at any
time is determined by a fractional size of the meristem
defined as

$$P = \frac{I_t}{I_s}$$

In Hall's work (1962) at 19°C the relevant cycle
was about 30 hours, so a fifth of a cell cycle would
be equivalent to a quarter of a day in hours. He assumes
that a fifth of the total population will divide and so
during this time the number of cells in the meristem
will be increased by a factor F where

$$F = 1 + \frac{1 - P}{5}$$

I_t is the total number of cells present at the beginning
of that interval. The value of I_t and therefore of P
is changing continuously, but its value at the beginning
of each time interval is assumed to apply throughout that
short interval.

The product of all the values of F is the factor by
which the number of integer cells on day 0 must be
multiplied to give the number present on day $10\frac{1}{4}$. Hall,
Lajtha and Oliver (1962) consider this a suitable end-
point for the calculation, because by the 10th day it
may be assumed that the growth rate is almost exclusively
due to the cells which are descendants of those which
retained their reproductive integrity at the time of
irradiation.

28.

A computer programme was written to find the fraction of cells surviving each dose (Hall, Lajtha and Oliver, 1962). This programme was modified and written for use on a Wang computor. A flow diagram for this programme appears in the Appendix B.

Model B.

An alternative model was proposed by Hall, Lajtha and Oliver (1962), in which it is assumed that all meristematic cells are preparing for division, but that the proportion of cells maintaining their reproductive integrity is proportional to the concentration of a specific substance, i.e. the fraction of those preparing for division is proportional to this concentration. It is also assumed that the maintenance of the reproductive integrity implies utilization of this substance in a given region or layer of cells and is proportional to the number of cells present which retain their reproductive integrity. Cells which have lost their reprodictive integrity due to lack of substance differentiate.

For this model, the growth rate as a fraction of that for a steady state population is given by

$$G = \frac{1.595P + e^{-1.595P} - 1}{0.7975}$$

P is the proportion of the total population. The increase in the fractional size of the meristem in a time equal to $\frac{1}{T}$th of the cell cycle is

$$F = 1 + \frac{1}{1.595TP} \left[2 - 2e^{-1.595P} - 1.595P \right]$$

Expanding this expression to the first two terms of
the exponential series gives (see Appendix C)

$$F = 1 + \frac{1 - 1.595P}{T}$$

This may be compared with the simple assumption

$$F = 1 + \frac{1 - P}{T} \qquad \text{derived in Model A.}$$

This model leads to a linear distribution of cells
within the cell cycle, and hence the simple fractions
of the cell cycle pertain. The step-by-step calculation
to compute the initial surviving fraction, f, is
essentially the same as in Model A. The computor
programme in Model B is more involved, however, because
there is no simple relationship between G and P. In
the programme an iterative procedure was used to
solve for P, (Hall, et al, 1962). This programme was
modified and written for use on a Wang computor.
A flow diagram for this programme appears in the Appendix.

Model C.

In this model, proposed by Oliver and Shepstone (1963),
the meristem is assumed fixed so that, as division takes
place, the excess cells are "squeezed out" of the
compartment and differentiate.

It was previously suggested (Hall, et al, 1962) that
this model would imply no differentiation during recovery
but if sterile cells remain in the compartment and count
towards the total until themselves extruded, the pattern

of reduced growth rate and slow recovery is to be
expected. The population in this instance is assumed
to be in exponential growth.

Model D.

In this model, brought forward by Dewey and Howard
(1963), an attempt is made to explain the dynamics of
the cells in the distal 2 mm of the root under standard
conditions. The presence of differentiating cells is
taken into account throughout the meristematic region.
A method to evaluate time parameters related to the
mitotic cycle of the cells is given in this model.

CHAPTER 4.

THE   VINCA   ALKALOIDS   AND   OTHER   CYTOTOXIC

AGENTS

CHAPTER 4.

THE VINCA ALKALOIDS AND OTHER

CYTOTOXIC AGENTS.

Introduction.

A phytochemical investigation of the Periwinkle
Vinca rosea Linn. has demonstrated that a number of
alkaloidal substances with antitumour activity can
be obtained from it.   Over 30 alkaloids have been
extracted, of which four - vinblastine, vinleurosine,
vincristine and vinrosidene are known definitely to
be active.

The two genera, Vinca and Catharanthus comprise
the group of plants referred to as the Periwinkle,
however, much confusion exists concerning the proper
nomenclature within these genera.

The Periwinkles are members of the alkaloid-rich
Apocynaceae. A paper by Bisset (1958) represents a
comprehensive review of the Apocynaceae.

Botanical Considerations.

Pichon (1951) consider the genus Catharanthus
to comprise six species of small shrubs and herbs
which are predominently indigenous to Madagaskar.
It spread to India, Indochina, Australia, South Africa
and to other countries.   It is a fast growing shrub,
woody at the base, 40 - 80 cms high, with erect branches.

The plant enjoyed a popular reputation in indigenous
medicine in various parts of the world.   Peckholt (1910)
described the use in Brazil of an infusion of the
leaves to control scurvy and haemorrhage, as a mouth-
wash for toothaches, and for the healing of chronic wounds.

The folklore reputation which the plant
enjoyed, independently stimulated its phytochemical
investigation in two different laboratories, unknown
to each other. One of the groups included Nobel,
Beer and Cutts at the Collis Laboratories in Ontario.
The other group included Svoboda, Johnson, Neuss
and Gorman in the Lilly Research Laboratories.
(Johnson, et al. 1963.)

Extractions from <u>Vinca rosea</u> Linn.

The Canadian group under Noble, Beer and Cutts
(1958) observed bone marrow depression in rats associated
with certain fractions when treated with extracts of
Vinca rosea. Continued investigations led to their
preparation of vincaleukoblastine, (V.L.B.) an alkaloid
capable of producing severe leukopenia in rats .
(Johnson et al, 1963). An extensive phytochemical
investigation resulted in the obtaining of leurosine,
an alkaloid closely related chemically to V.L.B., as
well as V.L.B. sulphate.(Svoboda, 1956).

It was shown that the activity of the alkaloids
of the leaves of Vinca rosea Linn were more active
than those contained in either the stem or roots.
(Johnson et al, 1963; Svoboda, 1956). The leaf
material was therefore used for the preparation of
different compounds and a procedure of differential
extractions was developed which separated the alkaloids
according to their basicities.

The structures of vinblastine, vincristine, and, to a lesser extent, vinleurosine, are reasonably well established. Modification of these large alkaloidal molecules is difficult. After making minor changes in the configuration of these alkaloids, marked differences in activity and side-effects have been observed, when treating mice with P1534 leukaemia.

Properties and Mode of Actions of a Few Drugs Extracted from _Vinca rosea_ Linn.

Of all the alkaloids extracted from _Vinca rosea_ Linn., vinleurosine, vincristine, vinblastine and vinrosidene have been found to be the most "active". Studies in _vivo_ and in _vitro_ have shown that these alkaloids have antitumour, antimitotic, stathmokinetic and toxic effects. These four properties are closely related and makes distinction between them difficult.

1. The Antimitotic Effects.

Vinblastine and vincristine, two closely related alkaloids, have been shown to be effective oncolytic agents. They cause an arrest of mitosis at the metaphase stage in a manner which may be similar to that of other mitotic poisons, such as colchicine and colcimid. They have been shown to cause dissolution of the mitotic spindle of _Pectinaria_ oöcytes. (Malawista, 1968). Polarized light and electron-microscopy was used to study the effects of various mitotic poisons on mitotic spindles.

2. <u>Stathmokinetic Properties</u>.

Studies of the stathmokinetic effects and other biological effects of vincristine on rats were performed by Frei <u>et al</u>. (1964). After a single dose of vincristine, an increase in the mitotic index in the marrow, duodenum and hair follicle of the rat was observed. In the bone marrow, this increase occured after 12 hours. Thereafter, the mitotic counts decreased rapidly. The increase in mitosis was found to be entirely due to the increase in the number of cells in metaphase.

The effects of vincristine on the bone marrow of five patients with malignant neoplastic diseases were studies. (Frei <u>et al</u>, 1964). In all five patients the M.I. increased sharply after single intravenous vincristine administrations, and a peak in M.I. occured after 12 hours. After 12 hours the M.I. decreased to normal.

Vincristine and vinblastine have been found to produce metaphase increase <u>in vivo</u> or <u>in vitro</u> in every mammalian system in which it has been studied. The mechanism of this stathmokinetic effect remains obscure. Although the morphological effects have been found to be indistinguishable from those produced by colchicine, the over-all biological effects of colchicine are dissimilar to those of the periwinkle alkaloids.

3. <u>Antitumour Studies</u>.

The most striking experimental biological effect
of the four <u>vinca</u> alkaloids, vinblastine, vincristine,
vinrosidene and vinleurosine, is their effectiveness
in prolonging life or, in some cases "curing" DBA/2
mice given implants of the P-1534 leukaemia. A
comparison of the anti-P-1534 activity of the four
compounds yielded the following results:
vinblastine, vincristine and vinrosidene resulted
in 100 per cent prolongation of leukaemia, whereas
a 50 - 100 per cent prolongation resulted after
vinleurosine treatment. A comparison of the
activities of the compounds on solid tumours has
been made as well. (Johnson, <u>et al</u>. 1963).

Vincristine was found to produce a complete
remission in 50 per cent patients with acute leukaemia,
(Karon, <u>et al</u>, 1962); objective tumour regression in
patients with Hodgkin's disease, lymphosarcoma, and
certain childhood solid tumours (Carobone <u>et al</u>. 1963;
Palmer, 1960; Armstrong, 1962). Vincristine has
produced definite, though limited benefit in patients
with carcinoma of the breast. (Armstrong, 1962).

4. <u>Toxic Effects</u>.

It was found that multiple intravenous doses of
vincristine and vinblastine caused marked leukopenia
in rats and dogs, causing death in some instances.
Toxicity studies with vincristine have also been
conducted in rabbits, monkeys, and cats. The acute

intravenous lethal dose for vincristine in mice
is approximately 2.0 mg/kg. Multiple doses of
vincristine of 0.1 mg/kg. caused death in some
instances. (Johnson, et al. 1963).

The major clinical toxic manifestations of
vincristine relate to the neuromuscular system,
the gastro-intestinal tract and the skin.
(Frei et al. 1964).

The relation between antitumour stathmokinetic
and toxic action of the vinca alkaloids remains
obscure. The stathmokinetic effects of vincristine
in vivo obtained by Cardinali (1963) are in good
agreement with the results obtained in vitro by
Palmer and Warren (1962). While vinblastine and
vincristine posess the same type of antimitotic
activity, they seem to differ quite markedly in
their antitumour effect. For instance, vincristine
sems to be active against acute lymphatic leukaemia,
(Costa, et al.1962; Karon, et al 1962; Rohn and Hodes,
1962; Palmer et al, 1962). Vinblastine, on the
other hand, seems to be of little use as an anti-
leukaemic agent. At present, the question of the
relationship between antitumour and antimitotic
effect of the two alkaloids mentioned above has no
definite answer. It is possible that the antitumour effect is completely independent of the
antimitotic effect, but it is also possible that
the two phenomena are more or less correlated.

<u>A Comparison of the Effects of X-Rays and</u>
<u>8-Ethoxycaffeine</u>.

Considerable work has been done on the effects of chemicals described as "radiomimetic" or "nucleotoxic" on the cells of broad bean meristems. Read and Gray (1959) have noted that a close parallel exists between the production of chromosome aberrations caused by ionizing x-rays and the gross effect on the growth of roots giving G_{min} and G_{10}. Meristematic cells of <u>Vicia</u> have been examined after ionizing radiation. It was found that the chromosomes appeared to be sticky and characteristic errors in spiralization have been observed (Darlington and La Cour, 1945). After the effects of stickiness had disappeared, the chromosomes appeared to be broken and out of line with each other.

Experiments on 8-Ethoxycaffeine (to be represented by E.O.C.) arose from the discovery by Kihlman and Levan (1949) that various purine derivatives could induct chromosome changes in root tips of the onion, <u>Allium cepa</u>. These changes appeared to be of the same kind as those produced by x-rays. In addition, mitosis was temporarily inhibited. Further similarities were that the production of chromosome aberrations by E.O.C. in <u>Allium</u> and in <u>Vicia</u> cells were influenced by

the concentration of dissolved oxygen in the
E.O.C. solutions.

After these discoveries were made by Kihlman
and Levan (1949), experiments on _Vicia_ seedlings
were conducted by Read and Gray (1959).

The effect of E.O.C. and x-rays on the root
meristem of _Vicia faba_ was shown to bear a
quantitative as well as a qualitative similarity.
Qualitatively, a comparison could be made of the
reduction of growth of seedlings after E.O.C.
treatment with the reduction in growth after
ionizing x-ray dosage. It was thus possible to
correlate E.O.C. treatment with x-ray treatment.
Quantitatively, by reducing the growth of two
groups of roots by the same degree, by an E.O.C.
treatment on the one hand, and by an x-ray
treatment on the other, it was found that the two
groups carried equal proportions of cells with
damaged chromosomes. (Read and Gray, 1959).

CHAPTER 5.

THE MODE OF ACTION OF DRUGS

ON RECEPTORS.

CHAPTER 5.

THE MODE OF ACTION OF DRUGS ON RECEPTORS.

INTRODUCTION.

The classical theories used to describe the relationship between the dose of a drug given and the response of a
tissue observed are all based on the law of mass action.
Approaches of this nature have been developed by Clark (1926),
Gaddum (1957), and Stephenson (1956). A "kinetic" theory
of drug action has been developed by Paton (1961, 1964). This
theory is based on the rate of drug-receptor combination.

A further theory, giving an analysis of the actions
of drugs and the relations between structure and action has
been developed (Ariëns 1964; Drill 1958). This theory of
dose-response relations for single drugs will be discussed
in this chapter.

THEORY.

When the effect of a drug is studied on a simple isolate
organ suspended in a bath fluid, the influence of drug
transference, transport, chemical transformation, excretion,
etc., is reduced to a minimum.

As a rule, the number of molecules added to the bath
fluid will be very large in comparison with the number of
molecules bound by the receptors. The specific receptors
are the counterpart of the drug molecules as far as the specif
interaction required for the induction of effect is concerned.

40.

The receptors may be molecules, parts of molecules or molecule complexes. A single receptor can be occupied by only one molecule of the drug at one time.

The formation of a drug-receptor complex may imply a very temporary interaction between drug-molecule and receptor: it may be just a slight contact between the drug molecule and the receptor. On the other hand, there may be a definite, possibly a prolonged, chemical binding between them.

The relation between a drug, A, and the receptor, R can be represented by:-

$$[R] \; + \; [A] \underset{k_2}{\overset{k_1}{\rightleftharpoons}} [RA] \qquad \qquad ....(5.1)$$

where $[R]$ is the concentration of free receptors,

$[A]$ is the drug concentration in the biophase, and

$[RA]$ is the concentration of the drug-receptor complex, that is, the quantity of drug bound to the specific receptors. The total concentration of receptors, $[r]$, is $[R] + [RA]$.

k_1 is the association rate constant,

k_2 is the dissociation rate constant .

Equation 5.1 represents a <u>reversible</u> interaction of drug molecules with receptors.

An increase in the concentration of the drug will result in an increase of the quantity of the drug-receptor complexes. Since the number of specific receptors in the biological object is limited, the maximal amount of drug-receptor complex has a limit, too. Increase of the concentration of the drug causes a saturation of the receptors. (Ariëns, 1964).

The arguments given below pertain as long as a gradual increase of the dose of the drug results in a gradual saturation of the receptor system.

In the case where the concentration of the drug is high compared with the number of specific receptors, it can be assumed to remain constant. Then the fraction of the total number of receptors, occupied by drug A, is represented by equation 5.2:

$$\frac{[RA]}{[r]} = \frac{1}{1 + (K_A / [A])} \qquad \dots.5.2$$

$$\text{where } K_A = \frac{k_2}{k_1}$$

$\frac{[RA]}{[r]}$ increases with concentration of the drug, [A] and decreases with the dissociation constant K_A of the drug-receptor complex RA. Thus, the "affinity" of the drug to the receptors is proportional to the reciprocal of K_A. E represents the effector cells.

In order to induce an effect, a drug must interact with the receptors, that is, it must have an "affinity" for the receptors. It must also interact with the receptors in an "effective" way; the drug must have an "intrinsic activity".

The effect of the drug will be proportional to the quantity of drug-receptor complexes formed. The proportionality constant, or the intrinsic activity of the drug is a measure of its ability to contribute to the stimulus, and thus to its effect.

42.

Let S_A be the stimulus, and S_M the maximum stimulus obtainable.

Thus,

$$\frac{S_A}{S_M} = \frac{\alpha}{(1 + (K_A/[A]))} \qquad \dots 5.3$$

where α represents the intrinsic activity of the drug.

If a linear proportionality between stimulus and effect is assumed, then the effect, E_A, induced in the effector, E, by a certain concentration of the drug, $[A]$, as a fraction of the maximal effect, E_m, obtainable with a drug, is represented by:

$$\frac{E_A}{E_m} = \frac{[RA]\,\alpha}{[R]} = \frac{\alpha}{1 + (K_A/[A])} \qquad \dots\dots 5.4$$

The effect obtained with a certain dose of A, that is, the activity of A in a general sense, increases with the intrinsic activity, α, and with the affinity, $\frac{1}{K_A}$. With high doses of A, the maximal effect for A, E_m, is reached and

$$\frac{E_A}{E_m} = \alpha$$

Further, $K_A = [A]$ if $E_A = \frac{1}{2} E_m$ (α taken as unity). $\dots 5.5$

This is thus a mathematical method for determining the values of the affinity and the intrinsic activity of the drug. The affinity is proportional to the reciprocal of that concentration of the drug, which gives a response equal to half of the maximal response obtainable with that drug. For a particular biological object and particular type of drug the intrinsic activity is proportional to the maximal effect obtainable with the drug in question. The intrinsic activity of the drug that gives the highest response is taken as unity; then, relative values for the intrinsic activity of other drugs can be given.

The dose-response curves as calculated from equation
5.4 are hyperbolas. On a log-dose scale they take the
character of sigmoid shaped curves. Fig. 5.1 represents
the theoretical dose-response curves calculated from
equation 5.4. The affinity as well as the intrinsic activity
are varied.

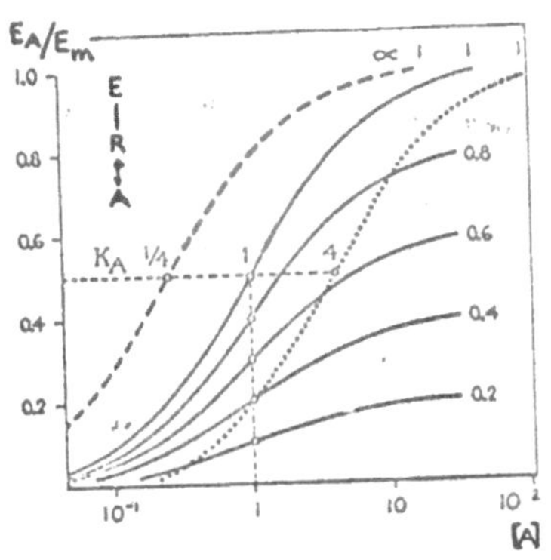

Fig. 5.1 Theoretical log concentration-
response curves for compounds with varying
values for the affinity ($1/K_A$) and the intrinsic
activity (α). Note the parallel shift in the
curves with a variation in K_A, and the decrease
in the maximal height and in the slope with a
decrease in α. (Concentration in M^{-1}).
(From Ariëns, E.J., 1964)

CHAPTER 6.

THE PROBLEM STATED

CHAPTER 6.

THE PROBLEM STATED.

Some effects of vincristine on the broad bean root
will be investigated.

(i) Vincristine is a known mitotic inhibitor and
by exposing seedlings to various doses of the drug, growth
patterns, similar to those resulting from x-irradiation
studies, ought to result.   As with radiation, survival
curves could then be obtained, using models, such as Model
A and B.   Such survival curves could then be compared to
those obtained by x-irradiation of _Vicia faba_. In this way
the dose of drug could be equated with x-ray dose.

(ii) Further, it ought to be possible to interpret
the action of vincristine on the root meristem of _Vicia
faba_ in terms of existing theories on the action of drugs
on tissue.   The survival curves obtained by using Models
A and B could again be compared to theoretical patterns
deduced from the existing drug laws.   In this way the
validity of the mathematical models could be further
tested, this time to a mode of action different to that
of radiation.

CHAPTER 7.

MATERIALS AND METHODS

MATERIALS and METHODS

The beans used for all experiments to be described
were of the hardy "Primo" variety, which stood up to
the radiation and vincristine treatments very well. In
experiments which involved the bean roots to be exposed
to aerobic and hypoxic solutions, the roots remained
unaffected by gas bubbling through the containers in
which they were emmersed.

Preparation of Seedlings for Experiments.

For each individual experiment, about 300 seedlings
of Vicia faba were used. The method of culture of the
beans was based on that used at the Medical Research
Council Radiobiological Research Unit, Harwell, (Evans,
Neary and Tonkinson, 1957; Read, 1959). This culture
method was used by Hall, Lajtha and Oliver (1962) as well.

Vicia seedlings were soaked in wet cottonwool in a
specially prepared lucite tray. They were moistened
daily for four days, or until the radicle just started
to appear.

The seedlings which had germinated were then carefully
planted, with the radicle pointing downwards, in moist
horticultural vermiculite, which was contained in a large
brass tank. The tank was kept at room temperature.
The vermiculite was autoclaved monthly at 126°C to remove
all fungi.

After four days the radicle had grown about 4 cms
in length. The seedlings were then carefully removed

from the vermiculite, washed, and their seed-coat
peeled off. Those that did not germinate, and all
damaged, abnormal or fungus infected beans were
discarded.

A cotyledon of each bean was numbered, and a
fudicial mark on the hypocotyl was made with permanent
black ink. This served as a reference point from which
the length of the bean root was measured.

The seedlings were then placed in the main culture
tank in fresh tap water for two days before the actual
experiment commenced. Two full cell cycles could thus
be completed under these conditions and the cell turn-
over in the meristem could thus reach equilibrium.

The culture tank was made from Perspex, and measured
70cm x 30cm x 30cm. A continuous flow of clear tap water
was passed into the tank at a rate of half a litre per
day. No nutrients were added to the water. With the
aid of a "Grant" temperature controller, the temperature
in the tank was kept constant at $25^{o}C \pm 0.5^{o}C$. A
propeller stirred the water continuously to maintain
circulation and ensured that the temperature was kept
uniform throughout the tank. Gray and Scholes (1951)
reported that a change of temperature of $1^{o}C$ resulted
in a 20 per cent change in the growth of the roots,
therefore meticulous control of the temperature was
needed.

A perspex tray with rows of holes, so that the
seedlings could pass through them easily, covered the
tank. The roots, suspended by the cotelydons, could
dangle freely in the water.

The plumules of the seedlings were removed as soon
as they appeared. Observations of previous experiments
have shown that there is a tendency for diurnal rythm in
mitotic index and root elongation throughout a twenty-
four hour period (Mottram 1913; Jüngling, etal 1930). In
order to eliminate this diurnal fluctuation, many
investigators remove the plumules and culture bean
seedlings in darkness. Evans (1964) found that, by
removing the plumules, the light effect of the growth is
eliminated.

After two days of growing in the main culture tank,
the seedlings were examined again. Those that showed any
signs of malformation were discarded - the rest were arranged
in groups of ten to twelve, depending on the nature of the
experiment. The groups consisted of beans of varying lengths
Lateral roots were removed as soon as they appeared.

<u>Preparation of Vincristine Solutions.</u>

Vincristine (oncovin) ampoules No. 649, containing 1 mg. oncovin and 10 mg. lactose, were obtained from Eli Lilly and Company, Indianapolis, U.S.A. (An accompanying ampoule of diluting solution was not used for the experiments to be described.   This solution contained 90 mg. sodium chloride, with 0.9 per cent benzyl alcohol as a preservative).

A series of experiments was conducted using different concentrations of vincristine for varying lengths of time.   Solutions of vincristine were made by dissolving the vincristine powder in appropriate amounts of distilled water, depending on the concentration required.   The solution was then transferred to small, flat, perspex jigs, which could hold up to 30 seedlings comfortably.   These jigs had gas inlets, so that nitrogen or medical air could pass through the solutions to create hypoxic or aerobic conditions.   A steady flow of gas was maintained through-out the treatment.   To keep the temperature of the solution constant during treatment, these perspex jigs were suspended in the main culture tank, (see Fig. 7.1).

After remaining in the drug for the desired length of time, the seedlings were washed, measured and returned to the culture tank.

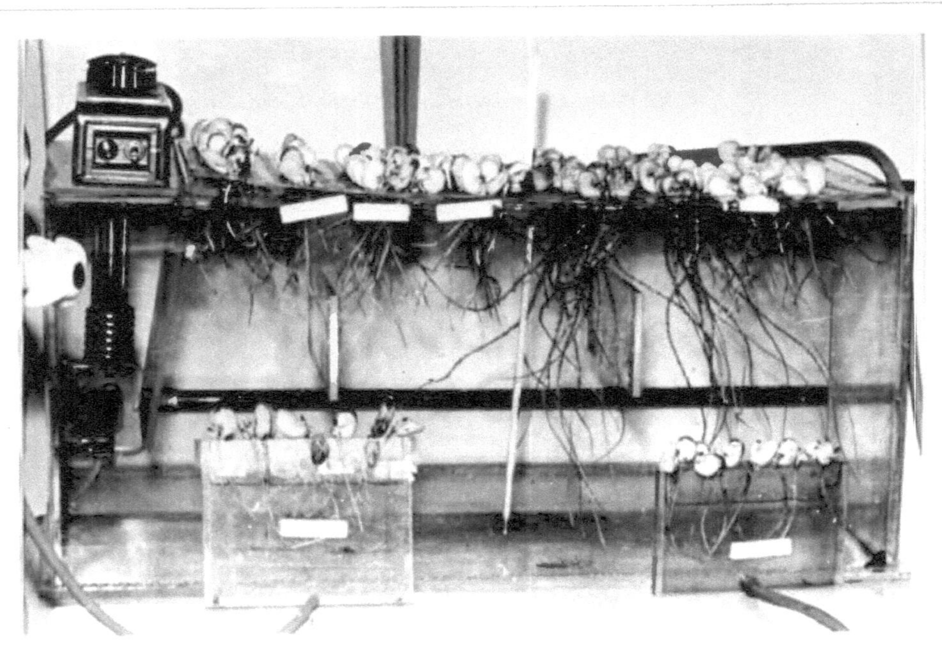

Fig. 7.1. The culture tank with the "Grant"
temperature controller. Seedlings to be
treated were emersed in flat perspex jigs
which contained vincristine solutions.

<u>Method of Irradiating</u>.

Seedlings to be irradiated were placed in a flat
perspex container, designed to hold about 30 seedlings
at a time. It was narrower at the bottom than the top,
so that the roots were congregated together and thus
were exposed to the same amount of radiation. This jig
measured 3 mm. deep in the direction of the beam of
radiation and 7 cm x 7 cm in cross section. It has a
gas inlet, through which medical air could be passed
to create aerobic conditions. This small container
could be slit into slots at one end of a 30 cm x 30 cm
x 30 cm perspex tank which was filled with water.

This tank was set up at 25 cm from the tube focus
with the long axis of the tank along the beam axis.

To measure the exact dose to the roots, a Baldwin
Farmer dosemeter was placed in a perspex holder and
slid into the treatment tank so that its centre coincided
with the centre of the volume occupied by the tips of the
roots during irradiation, (see Fig. 7.2).

The time taken to deliver 50 R was measured and the
dose rate in rads per minute was computed using corrections
for temperature and pressure, and using the appropriate
Roentgen to rad conversion factor. (This factor was that
recommended by the International Commission for Radio-
logical Units, 1962). After the times to deliver the
doses to the seedlings had been computed, the chamber
was removed, and its holder was exchanged for the one
to hold the <u>Vicia</u> seedlings.

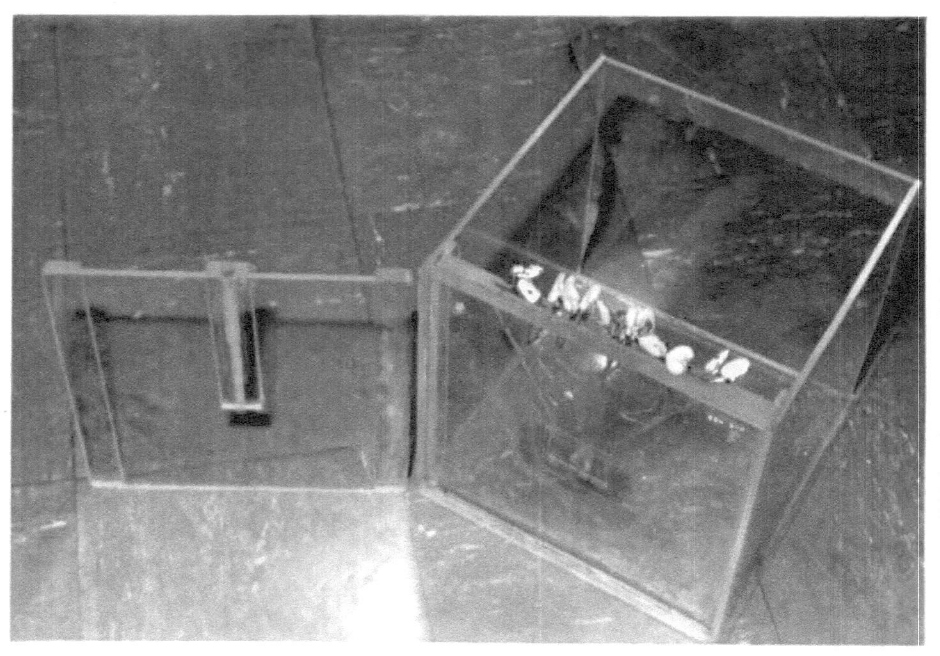

Fig. 7.2   Perspex tank which was used for
           irradiating purposes.   On the left
           is the perspex holder to accomodate
           a Baldwin Farmer dosemeter.

Both jig and tank were filled with tap water. Each
group of beans to be irradiated was transferred in turn
to the jig, and medical air was passed through the water
during exposure and for fifteen minutes beforehand.
This is sufficient time for equilibrium to be reached
between oxygen tension of the water and the tissue of
the root (Read 1952). Precautions were taken to
ensure that the water level in the tank and jig remained
constant.

The x-ray machine used to irradiate the seedlings
was a Philips 250/25 Therapy Unit, operated at 250 k.Vp
and 15 mA. The beam was filtered through 0.25 mm copper,
0.8 mm Sn and 1.0 mm Al filters. A 20 cm x 20 cm
applicator was used to cover the volume occupied by
the root tips adequately. During the irradiation of
any group, the tube voltage and tube current were
maintained by using the manual controls.

The group of seedlings to be irradiated were arranged
in the jig with their roots sloping towards the centre of
the funnel, the longer roots being placed towards the out-
side. The tube head was adjusted to ensure that all roots
were in the uniform part of the field.

Gray and Scholes (1951) found that the root tip was
sensitive to radiation, and that irradiation of the
remainder of the root does not affect subsequent growth
of the primary root. The cotelydons were, however,
shielded from radiation with the aid of lead strips (see
Fig. 7.3.).

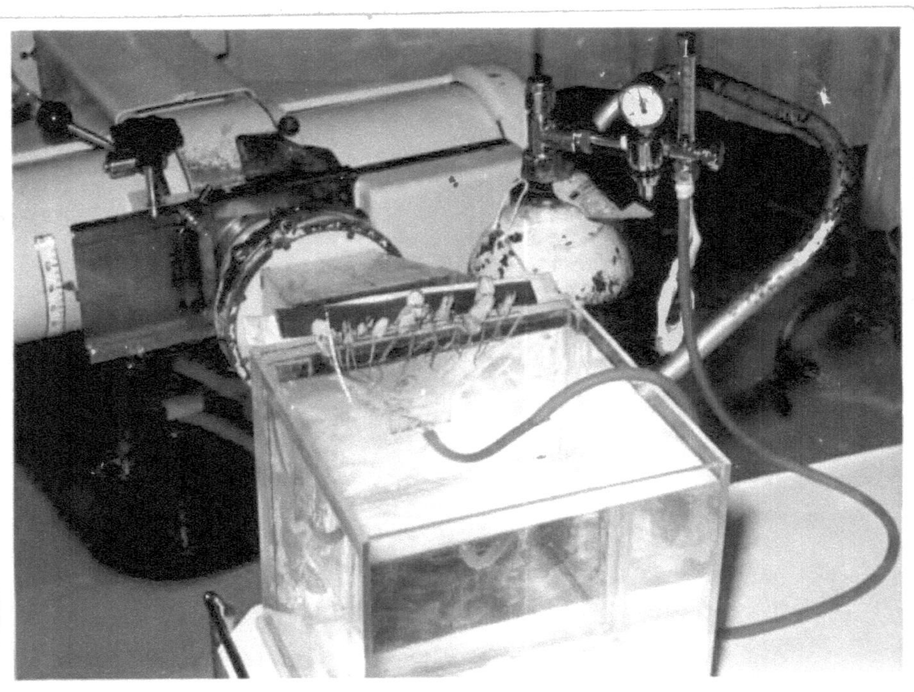

Fig. 7.3. Perspex jig set up in front of x-ray
machine. Seedlings were aerated by passing medical air
through the tank.

<u>Macroscopic Method for Assessing Damage by Radiation</u>
<u>and Vincristine.</u>

Individual roots vary considerably in both growth
rate and response to radiation and drugs. Consequently,
groups of between nine and fifteen roots were exposed
to each treatment and the results were treated by
statistical methods. The statistical methods are
described in the appendix A.

After an exposure to ionizing radiation, the growth
rate of the roots is reduced to a degree which depends
on the size of the dose. A large dose may cause a
progressive reduction to zero, and the root, which turns
brown, may not grow again. In some cases a white cone
appears at the tip, and growth is resumed as a thin thread.
After smaller doses the growth rate may not reach zero.
There is a minimum growth rate after four days, followed
by a recovery. The growth rate may eventually exceed
that of the controlls, but the roots are thinner.

The roots of seedlings treated with vincristine
react in a similar way. The growth rate is reduced,
depending on the concentration of, and length of exposure
to the drug. Again, a large dose may cause a progressive
reduction in the growth rate to zero. After smaller doses,
a minimum growth rate after four days, followed by a
recovery is observed. Some of the treated roots, however,
become hard and stubby, whereas, after very severe doses,
roots tend to become very soft, jellyish and difficult to
handle without damaging them. Some root tips had a

55.

tendency to corkscrew - this made the measuring of
them rather inaccurate.

The control groups, as well as the treated beans
were measured on day O as well as each day following
experimentation for eleven days. Reasons for making
these measurements will be given later in this section.
Measurements of the groups took place at roughly the
same time each day.

The measurements of the beans were made as follows:-
a meter rule was placed along the length of the culture
tank. The beanroot to be measured was carefully removed
from the tank and placed along the rule. The reference
mark just below the cotelydon was placed opposite the
"O" mark on the rule, the root was carefully straightened,
and its length to the tip measured.

Lateral roots were removed, the plumules cut off,
and after measurement, the seedling was placed into its
position in the culture tank.

Gray and Scholes (1951) have reported that the
lifting and measuring of the bean root did not affect the
growth of the root.

It was found that the growth increment of the control
group was not contant, and that it declined towards the
eigth day. Thus the beans had to be measured daily, and
their growth increment calculated as a fraction of the
growth increment of the control group measured on the
same day. Pilet (1961) offers a possible explanation
for this decrease in control growth: a root hormone,

auxin, inhibits growth. It is thought that auxin
inhibits growth more in older tissue than in younger.
Thus it can be expected that growth rate falls as the
root ages.

From the daily growth increments of the treated
beans, curves were drawn, correcponding to each dose,
to show the "daily growth" as a function of the control
group. This increment in growth was regarded as that
pertaining to a time halfway between the times at which
the measurements were made.

In general, three parameters have been used by
various workers to score the effect of radiation on
root growth:

a) The 'mean lethal dose' - defined to be the dose
    which results in cessation of growth for four or
    more days by half the roots of the group.
    (Gray and Scholes, 1951;Spalding, Langham and
    Anderson, 1956, 1958).

b) The 'minimum growth rate' of the root, reached
    four to five days after irradiation and expressed
    as a fraction of the control roots of the same
    length (Gray and Scholes, 1951) or as a fraction
    of roots of the same age (Lajtha, Hall and
    Oliver, 1962). This quantity is marked G min
    in Fig. 7.4.

c) The 'growth in ten days' - defined to be the mean
    increment in lengths of the irradiated roots in
    ten days following irradiation, expressed as a

fraction of control roots in the same period

(Read, 1952). It is, in effect, the area under the curve up

to the tenth day in Fig. 7.4

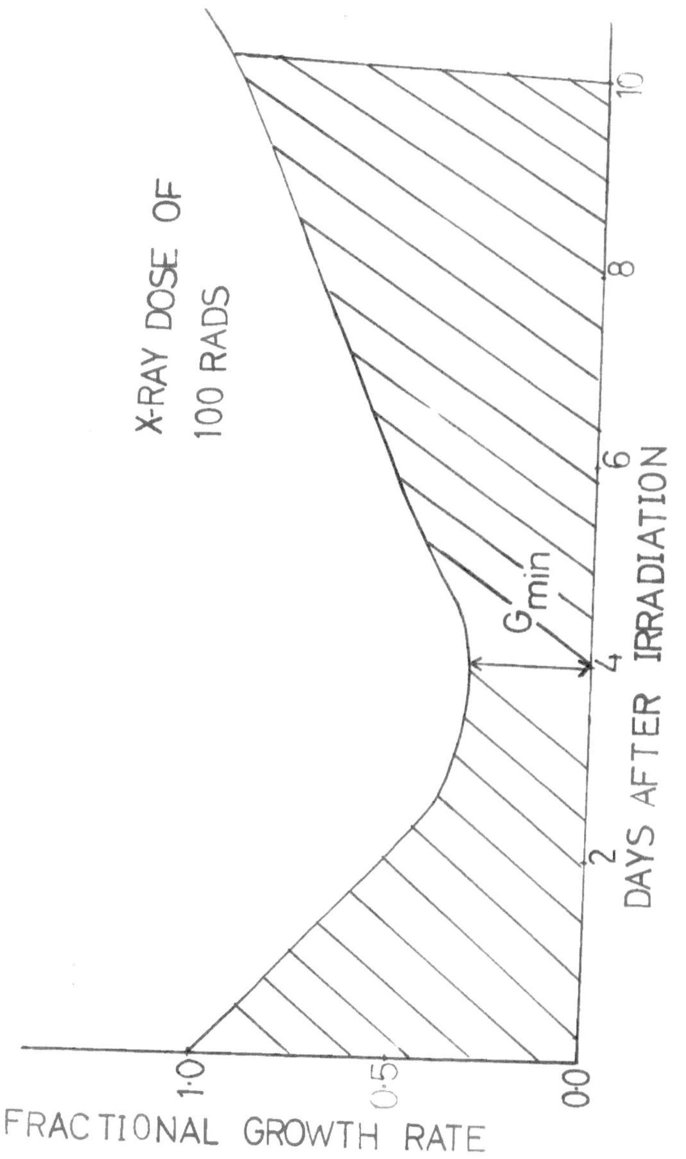

Fig.7.4. Fractional growth rate of seedlings after 100 rads
x-irradiation. G_{10} is the area under the curve up
to the tenth day (shaded).

59.

CHAPTER 8.

RESULTS

CHAPTER 8.

RESULTS.

<u>Experiment 1.</u>

<u>The response of Vicia faba seedlings to x-irradiation.</u>

Following the method of irradiation and
measurements described in Chapter 7, doses of
50, 100, 150, 200 and 250 rads were given
respectively to five groups of fifteen roots
per group. On surveying the literature on
irradiation doses to <u>Vicia</u> seedlings, it was
found that doses in the range 50 - 250 rads caused
adequate reduction in the growth rate of the roots.
Doses greater than 250 rads proved to be too severe
for recovery to take place. (Gray and Scholes 1951;
Hornsey, S. 1956; Hall and Lajtha, 1963; Hall, 1961).

The relevant growth curves are given in Fig. 8.1.
The values of G_{10} and G_{min} are given in Table 8.1.

Using Model A and Model B separately, the
fraction of cells surviving radiation damage was
calculated. The factor F, by which the number of
cells in the meristem increases has been calculated
for each $\frac{1}{4}$ day (corresponding to one-fifth of the
cell cycle). Using this factor, the surviving
fraction F has been calculated. As an example,
the data for 50 rads using the two models is given
in Table 8.2 and 8.3. This calculation was repeated
for each dose. Table 8.4 gives the fraction surviving

60.

the single acute doses of radiation, using
Models A and B. Fig. 8.2 shows the dose
response curve for <u>Vicia</u> using the two models.

The standard deviation on the fraction of
cells surviving 50 rads using Model A was
calculated by reading the maximum values of
the fractional growth and finding the corresponding
fraction of cells surviving. This was repeated
using the lowest figures of fractional growth.
A maximum deviation of 0.14 was found.
It is shown in Fig. 8.2.

Table 8.1.

Dose (rads)	G_{min}	G_{10}
50	0.579 ± 0.11	0.775 ± 0.12
100	0.35 ± 0.04	0.58 ± 0.14
150	0.178 ± 0.02	0.376 ± 0.12
200	0.148 ± 0.02	0.228 ± 0.12
250	0.11 ± 0.02	0.173 ± 0.12

TABLE 8.2

Data for 50 rads, using Model A.

Time (days)	$\sqrt{G}=P=\dfrac{I_t}{I_s}$	Factor F**	Product
.00	1.0000	1.0000	1.0000
.25	0.9273	1.0145	1.0145
.50	0.8246	1.0350	1.0501
.75	0.8000	1.0400	1.0921
1.00	0.7874	1.0425	1.1385
1.25	0.7745	1.0450	1.1898
1.50	0.7681	1.0463	1.2480
1.75	0.8246	1.0350	1.2887
2.00	0.8000	1.0400	1.3402
2.25	0.7874	1.0425	1.3972
2.50	0.7615	1.0476	1.4639
2.75	0.8306	1.0338	1.5134
3.00	0.8366	1.0326	1.5629
3.25	0.8660	1.0267	1.6048
3.50	0.9000	1.0200	1.6368
3.75	0.8831	1.0233	1.6751
4.00	0.8602	1.0279	1.7219
4.25	0.8366	1.0326	1.7782
4.50	0.8246	1.0350	1.8405
4.75	0.8366	1.0326	1.9007
5.00	0.8602	1.0279	1.9538
5.25	0.8831	1.0233	1.9995
5.50	0.8944	1.0211	2.0417
5.75	0.8888	1.0222	2.0871
6.00	0.8831	1.0233	2.1358
6.25	0.8717	1.0256	2.1906
6.50	0.8717	1.0256	2.2468
6.75	0.8944	1.0211	2.2942
7.00	0.9219	1.0156	2.3300
7.25	0.9486	1.0102	2.3540
7.50	0.9539	1.0092	2.3756
7.75	0.9273	1.0145	2.4102
8.00	0.9165	1.0166	2.4504
8.25	0.8888	1.0222	2.5049
8.50	0.8660	1.0267	2.5720
8.75	0.8955	1.0211	2.6263
9.00	0.9327	1.0134	2.6616
9.25	0.9539	1.0092	2.6862
9.50	0.9746	1.0050	2.6998
9.75	0.9746	1.0050	2.7134
10.00	0.9746	1.0050	2.7272
10.25	0.9746	1.0050	2.7410

** Factor F, by which number of cells in meristem is increased during $\tfrac{1}{4}$ day. $F = 1 + \dfrac{1 - P}{5}$

62.

If f is the initial fraction surviving radiation,
then f I_s is the number of integer cells in the meristem
on day 0, and 2.7410 fI_s is the number on day 10.25.
From the second column it is known that on day 10.25,
$\frac{I_t}{I_s}$ = 0.9746. Therefore the total number of cells
present is 0.9746 I_s.

These two qualities can now be equated:

$$2.7410 \; fI_s = 0.9746 \; I_s$$

$$\therefore \; f = 0.36$$

Time (Days)	P'	F	Product of F's
0.00	1.000000	0.9998	0.9998
0.25	.910617	1.0109	1.0108
0.50	.788641	1.0276	1.0387
0.75	.760987	1.0316	1.0716
1.00	.745925	1.0338	1.1079
1.25	.732098	1.0359	1.1378
1.50	.724567	1.0371	1.1904
1.75	.788641	1.0276	1.2233
2.00	.760987	1.0316	1.2620
2.25	.745925	1.0338	1.3048
2.50	.717037	1.0383	1.3548
2.75	.796172	1.0265	1.3907
3.00	.802469	1.0256	1.4263
3.25	.836419	1.0208	1.4561
3.75	.857777	1.0179	1.5050
4.00	.830123	1.0217	1.5377
4.25	.802469	1.0256	1.5771
4.50	.788641	1.0276	1.6206
4.75	.802469	1.0256	1.6622
5.00	.830123	1.0217	1.6983
5.25	.857777	1.0179	1.7287
5.50	.870370	1.0162	1.7568
5.75	.874074	1.0170	1.7868
6.00	.857777	1.0179	1.8189
6.25	.843950	1.0198	1.8549
6.50	.843950	1.0198	1.8917
6.75	.870370	1.0162	1.9224
7.00	.903086	1.0119	1.9454
7.25	.935802	1.0077	1.9604
7.50	.942098	1.0069	1.9741
7.75	.910617	1.0109	1.9957
8.00	.896790	1.0127	2.0211

Cont. overleaf.

Table 8.3 (Cont.)

Time (Days)	P'	F	Product of F's
8.25	.864074	1.0170	2.0557
8.50	.836419	1.0208	2.0985
8.75	.870370	1.0162	2.1326
9.00	.916913	1.0101	2.1543
9.25	.942098	1.0069	2.1693
9.50	.968518	1.0036	2.1773
9.75	.968518	1.0036	2.1853
10.00	.968518	1.0036	2.1934
10.25	.968518	1.0036	2.1934

From equation C6 in Appendix C,

$$G = 1.595 \ P^2,$$

G has been calculated and plotted in terms of P.

Taking experimentally observed values of G for the meristem, the corresponding values of P and hence of F, have been read off the graph to give the factors of increase in the meristem population.

From Table 8.3, the product of all the F factors is 2.1934. From the graph, the population as a fraction of the control population at $10\frac{1}{4}$ days corresponding to a growth factor (G) of 0.94, is 0.8. Thus the initial fraction (f) of the population surviving a dose of 100 rad is given by :

$$f = \frac{0.94}{2.1934}$$

$$f = 0.43$$

<u>Table 8.4.</u>

Comparison of the fraction of cells surviving
radiation dosage, using Model A and Model B.

Dose (rads)	Model A	Model B
50	$0.3556^{\pm}0.14$	0.43
100	0.1350	0.198
150	0.0458	0.09
200	0.0078	0.0121
250	0.001	0.001

Straight line regressions were fitted to the
data (on the exponential portion of the graph)
by the method of least squares. This was done for
both models. The slopes of the graphs, as well as
the intercepts on the Y-axis, could then be
calculated. The results appear in Table 8.5.
The straight line regression on Model A values is
shown in Fig. 8.2.

<u>Table 8.5.</u>

Dosage (rads)	Fraction Surviving	
	Model A	Model B
50	0.416	0.552
100	0.121	0.173
150	0.035	0.051
200	0.010	0.017
Intercept on Y-axis	1.4	1.8
Slope of line	-0.25	-0.02

37 per cent dose slope : 40 rads.

The 37 per cent dose slope was read off the graph
(see Fig. 8.2) and was found to be 40 rads.   This corresponds to the dose required to reduce the surviving fraction
to e^{-1} of its original value.

As in chapter 5, let E_A = the effect induced by the
effector, E, i.e. the number of cells "hit".

Let E_m = maximal effect obtainable.

Then : Fraction of cells hit $= \dfrac{E_A}{E_m}$

And   : Fraction of cells surviving $= \dfrac{E_m - E_A}{E_m}$

$$= 1 - \dfrac{E_A}{E_m}$$

$\therefore$ Fraction of cells "hit" $= 1 -$ Fraction of cells surviving

Table 8.6 gives the fraction of cells hit for various
radiation dosages.

TABLE 8.6

Dose (Rads)	Fraction surviving.	(1 – Fraction surviving)	
		Model A	Model B
10	1.0	0	0
50	0.416	0.584	0.57
100	0.121	0.879	0.802
150	0.035	0.965	0.91
200	0.010	0.990	0.999

Fig 8.3 depicts the effect of radiation, E_A, as a fraction of the maximal effect, F_m , against $\log_{10}$ of the radiation dose. The "relative affinity" of the radiation to Vicia seedlings , i.e. $1/K_A$ was found to be $1/40$ $(\text{rads})^{-1}$.

Experiment 2.

<u>The response of Vicia faba seedlings to vincristine.</u>

Preliminary experiments with vincristine were carried out to obtain suitable methods of application of the drug to <u>Vicia</u> seedlings and to determine which concentration - time relations would apply to radio-biological studies. Treatments using 1 mg vincristine/ 10 ml water proved to be too severe for recovery of the seedlings to take place.

Dose-response curves were obtained using 1 mg vincristine dissolved in 40 ml water for 0.5, 0.75, 1, 1.5, 2, 2.5 and 3 hours. For each treatment time 15 seedlings were used. A group of 20 untreated seedlings served as controls. The method of drug application has been described in Chapter 7. After treatment with vincristine, the seedlings were returned to the culture tank (kept at 25°C) and were measured daily for 11 days.

The daily growths of the seedlings appears in Fig. 8.4. The fraction of cells surviving each dose was calculated by using Model A. The standard deviation on the fraction of cells surviving 1mg/40 ml for 0.75 hours was calculated, and found to be 0.1. (The method of this calculation has been discussed in Experiment 1, on the standard deviation on the fraction of cells surviving 50 rads).

The experiment was repeated, using the same concentration-time relations as in the previous experiment.   The fraction of cells surviving each dose was calculated using Model A. The two experiments will be referred to as Exp. 2(a) and 2(b) respectively.   The results of these experiments appear in Table 8.7, and Fig. 8.5

<u>Table 8.7</u>

Fraction of cells surviving vincristine (1 mg/40 ml) using Model A.

Time (hours)	Percent conc. x time x 10^{-3}	Fraction surviving	
		Exp. 2(a)	Exp. 2(b)
0.50	1.25	0.7200	0.3800
0.75	1.85	0.25±0.1	0.1500
1.00	2.50	0.005	0.0049
2.00	5.00	0.0040	0.003
3.00	7.50	0.0025	0.0025
Intercept on Y-axis:		30.20	41.41
Slope:		-0.70	-0.87

The unit of "dose" used turns out to be the product of the percentage concentration and the time in hours.   This product is expressed in the results as a decimal fraction without units.

The 37 per cent dose slope on the initial exponential portion of Fig. 8.5 was found to be 0.2 x 10^{-3}.   This corresponds to a period of 4.8 minutes of exposure to the drug.

Experiment 3:-

A comparative study, using 1 mg/80 ml was carried
out for 0.5, 1, 1.5, 2, 3, 4, 6, 8 and 10 hours. In this
case, both Models A and B were used to compute the fraction
of cells surviving each dose.   The values appear in
Table 8.8.

Fig. 8.5 shows the dose-response curves obtained
when seedlings were exposed to 1 mg/40 ml as well as 1
mg/80 ml for varying lengths of time.   Straight line
regressions were fitted to the exponential portions of the
survival curves by the method of least squares. From these,
the intercepts on the Y-axis as well as the 37 per cent
dose slope could be calculated.   The values are given in
Tables 8.7 and 8.8.

Fig. 8.6 shows the fraction of cells surviving doses
of 1 mg/80 ml, using Models A and B.

Table 8.8

Fraction of cells surviving doses of vincristine (1mg/80 ml)
using Models A and B.

Time (hours)	Per cent conc. x time ($\times 10^{-3}$)	Fraction surviving	
		Model A	Model B
1	1.25	0.310	0.110
1.5	1.87	0.025	0.030
2	2.50	0.005	0.005
4	5.00	0.0051	0.0051
6	7.50	0.0033	0.0030
8	10.0	0.0035	0.0030
10	12.50	0.0025	0.0020
Slope:		-0.80	-0.82
Intercept on Y-axis:		35.60	36.0

The 37 per cent dose slope on the initial exponential
portion of the graph (Fig. 8.6) was found to be 0.2×10^{-3},
which corresponds to a period of 9 minutes of exposure to
the drug.

Experiment 4:-

Vicia seedlings were exposed to various concentratio
of vincristine for a fixed period of time.
The concentrations that were applied were:

1 mg / 80 ml for 1 hour
1 mg / 40 ml for 1 hour
1 mg / 20 ml for 1 hour
1 mg / 10 ml for 1 hour.

The daily growth curves for these groups of seedling
appear in Fig. 8.7

Table 8.9 gives the fraction of cells surviving the
doses (using Model A):-

Table 8.9

Drug concentration	per cent conc. x time	Fraction surviving
1 mg/80 ml	1.25×10^{-3}	0.42
1 mg/40 ml	2.5×10^{-3}	0.10
1 mg/20 ml	5.0×10^{-3}	0.04
1 mg/10 ml	10.0×10^{-3}	0.01

<u>Drug Effect.</u>

As in Chapter 5, let E_A represent the effect of the drug of concentration $[A]$. Let E_m represent the maximum effect obtainable with the drug. i.e. all the cells occupied.

Then: Fraction of cells "hit" $= \dfrac{E_A}{E_m}$

and Fraction of cells surviving $= \dfrac{E_m - E_A}{E_m}$

$\therefore$ Fraction of cells "hit" $= 1 -$ Fraction of cells surviving.

Table 8.10 shows the variation of E_A/E_m with different dosages of vincristine. (The concentration was kept constant, i.e. 1 mg/40 ml, but the time of exposure to the drug was varied. Data from experiment 2(b)).

<u>Table 8.10</u>

per cent conc. x time x 10^{-3}	Fraction surviving (Model A)	1 - Fraction surviving
1.20	0.3800	0.6200
1.85	0.1500	0.8500
2.50	0.0049	0.9951
5.00	0.0030	0.9970
7.50	0.0025	0.9975

Table 8.11 shows the variation of E_A/E_m with different
dosages of vincristine (The concentration was kept constant
i.e. 1 mg/80 ml, but the time of exposure to the drug
was varied. Data from Experiment 3).

Table 8.11

per cent conc. x time x 10^{-3}	Fraction surviving (Model A)	1 - Fraction surviving
1.25	0.310	0.690
1.87	0.025	0.975
2.50	0.005	0.995
5.00	0.0051	0.995
7.50	0.0033	0.9967
10.00	0.0035	0.9965
12.50	0.0025	0.9975

Table 8.12 gives the variation of E_A/E_m with different
dosages. (Here the time of exposure to the drug was kept
constant, i.e. for one hour, while the concentration of
the vincristine was varied. Data from Exp. 4)

Table 8.12

per cent conc. x time x 10^{-3}	Fraction surviving (Model A)	1 - Fraction surviving
1.25	0.42	0.58
2.50	0.10	0.90
5.0	0.04	0.96
10.0	0.010	0.99

Figure 8.8 shows the log dose-response curve. The data
has been taken from Tables 8.10, 8.11 and 8.12.

The "affinity" of the drug to the receptors, i.e.
$\frac{1}{K_A}$ was found to correspond to a vincristine dose of
$\frac{1}{10^{-3}}$ i.e. 10^{+3}.

Because drug dosage is expressed as a decimal fraction without
units, the "affinity" of the drug is also expressed without
units. (The affinity is proportional to the reciprocal of
that concentration of the drug that gives a response equal
to half the maximal response obtainable with the drug).

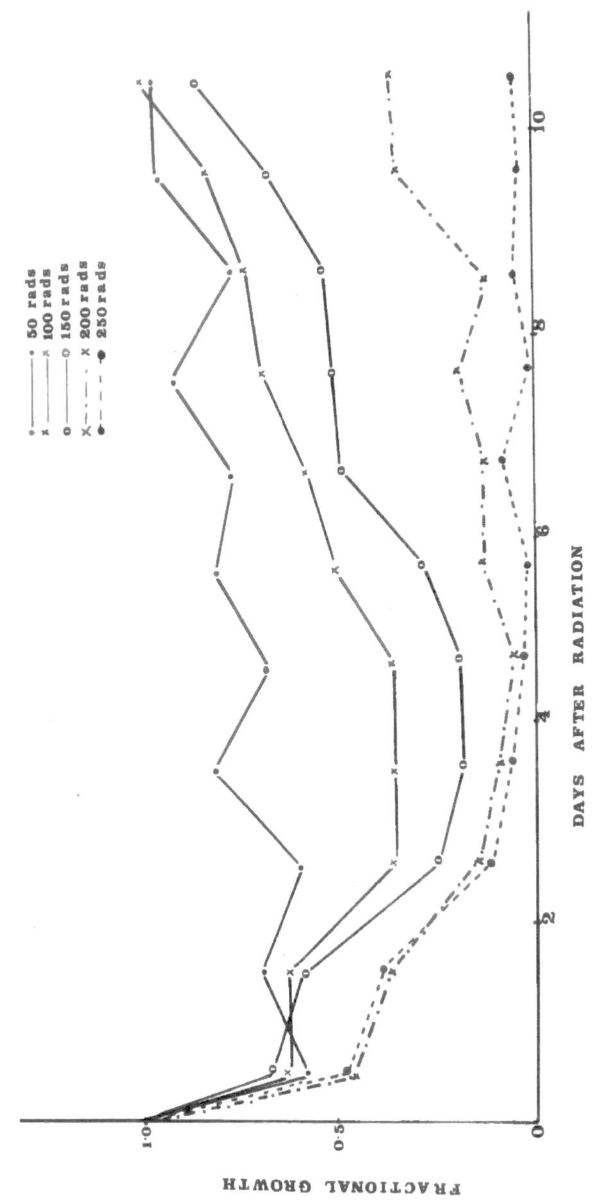

Fig. 8.1. Ordinate: Growth rate, after various doses of x-irradiation, expressed as a fraction of that for controls of equal age.

Abscissa: days after irradiation. (Exp.1)

77.

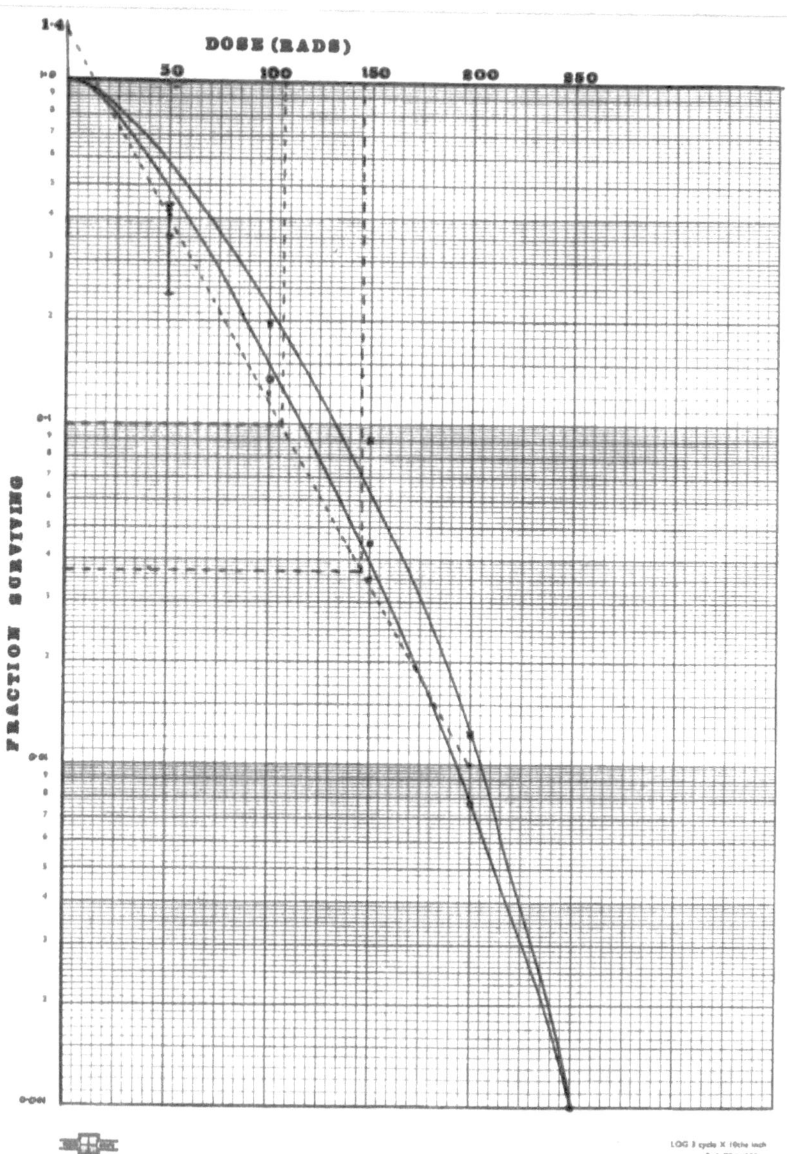

Fig. 8.2   Fraction of cells surviving radiation dosages.(Exp.1).

●————● (Model A)

x————x (Model B)

Dotted line: least squares fit to Model A.

The 37% dose slope yields a dose of 40 rads.

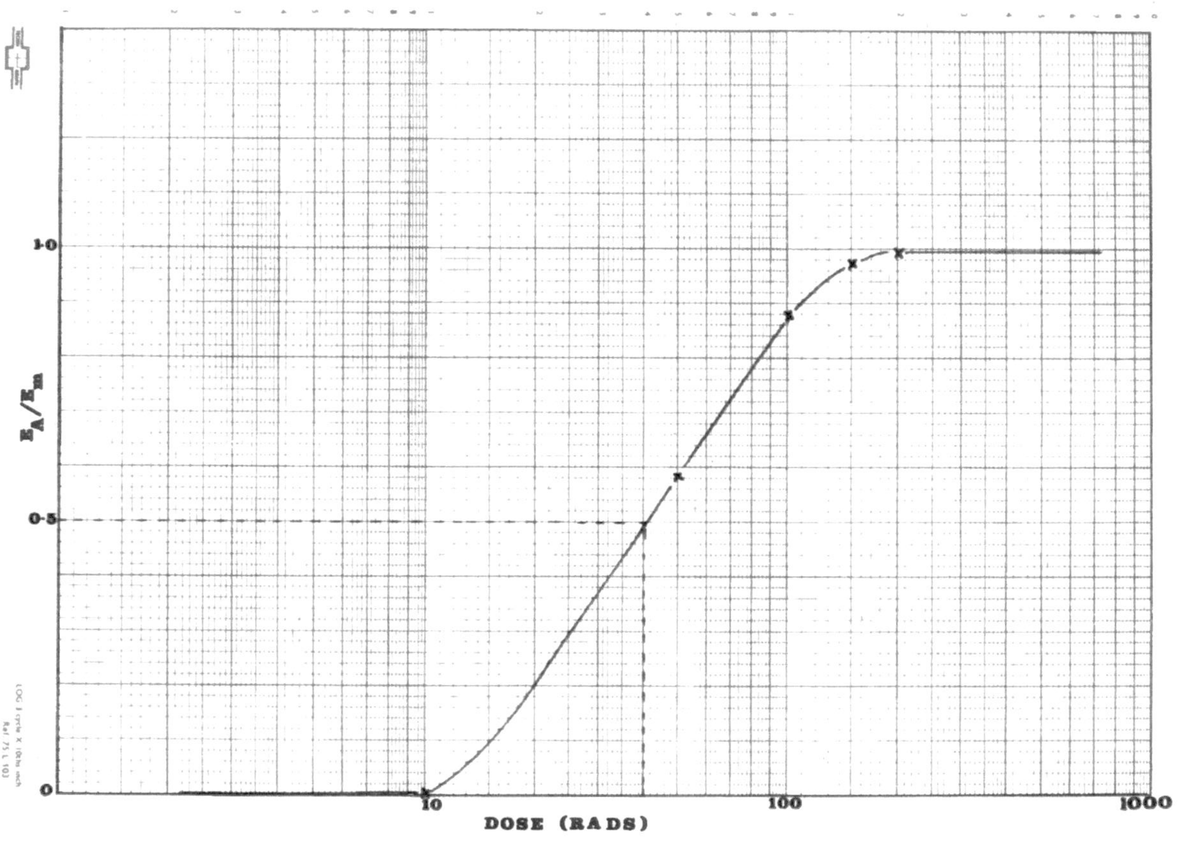

Fig. 8.3. Log-concentration response of <u>Vicia</u> seedlings to radiation. The "relative affinity",

$$1/\ K_A = \frac{1}{40}\ (rads)^{-1}$$

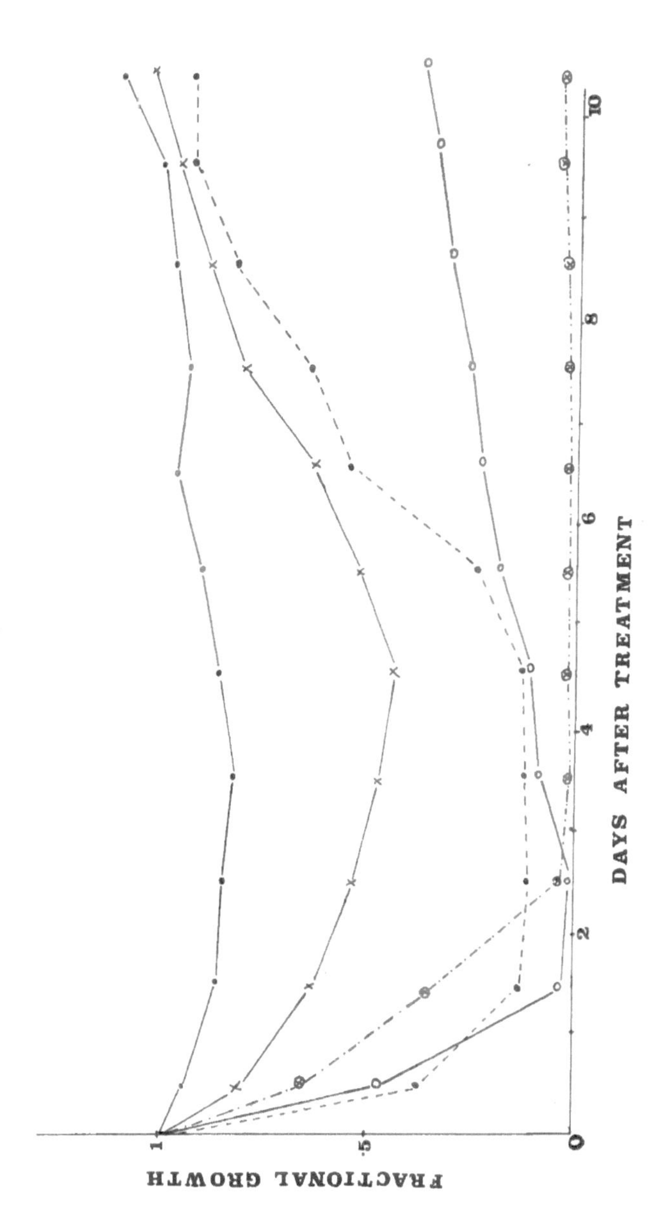

Fig. 8.4: Ordinate: Fractional growth of _Vicia_ seedlings after exposure to vincristine (1 mg/40 ml) for various lengths of time. Abscissa: Days after treatment. (Exp.2).

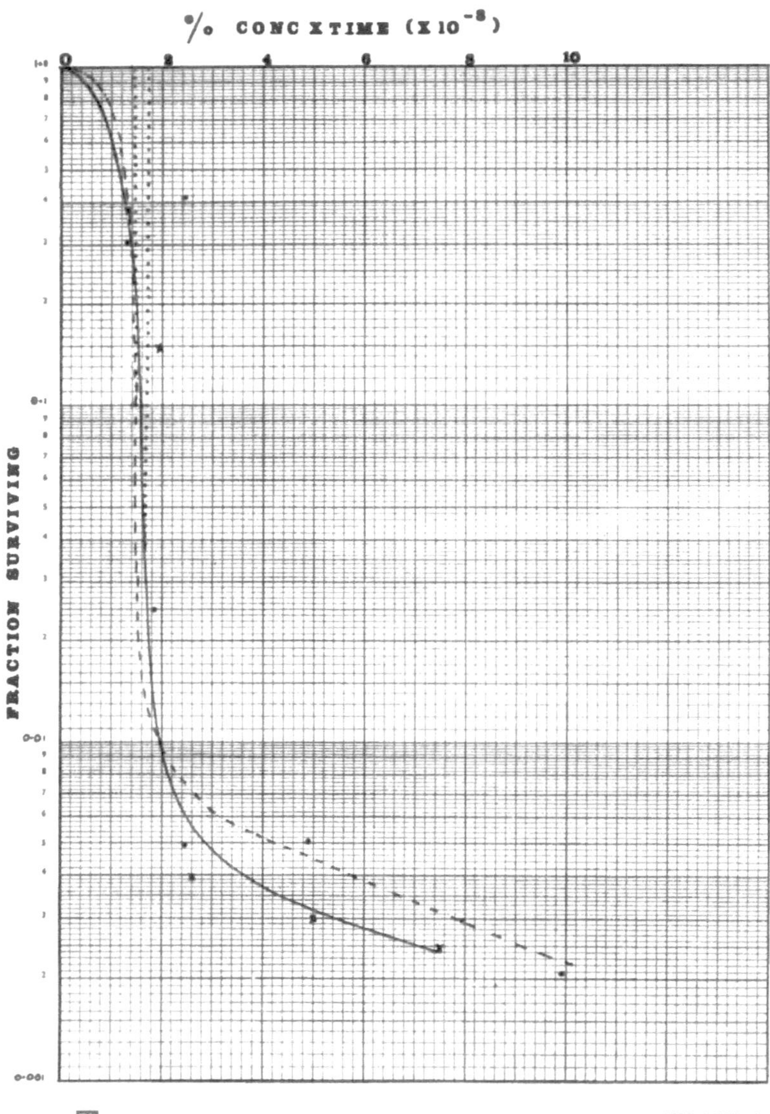

Fig. 8.5: Fraction of cells surviving vincristine doses
(Using Model A.)

x——x 1 mg/40 ml (Exp. 2(b))
•------• 1 mg/80 ml (Exp. 3)

The 37% dose slope: 0.2×10^{-3}, i.e. 4.5 minutes of
exposure to the drug (1 mg/40 ml) and 9 minutes of
exposure (1 mg/80 ml).

81.

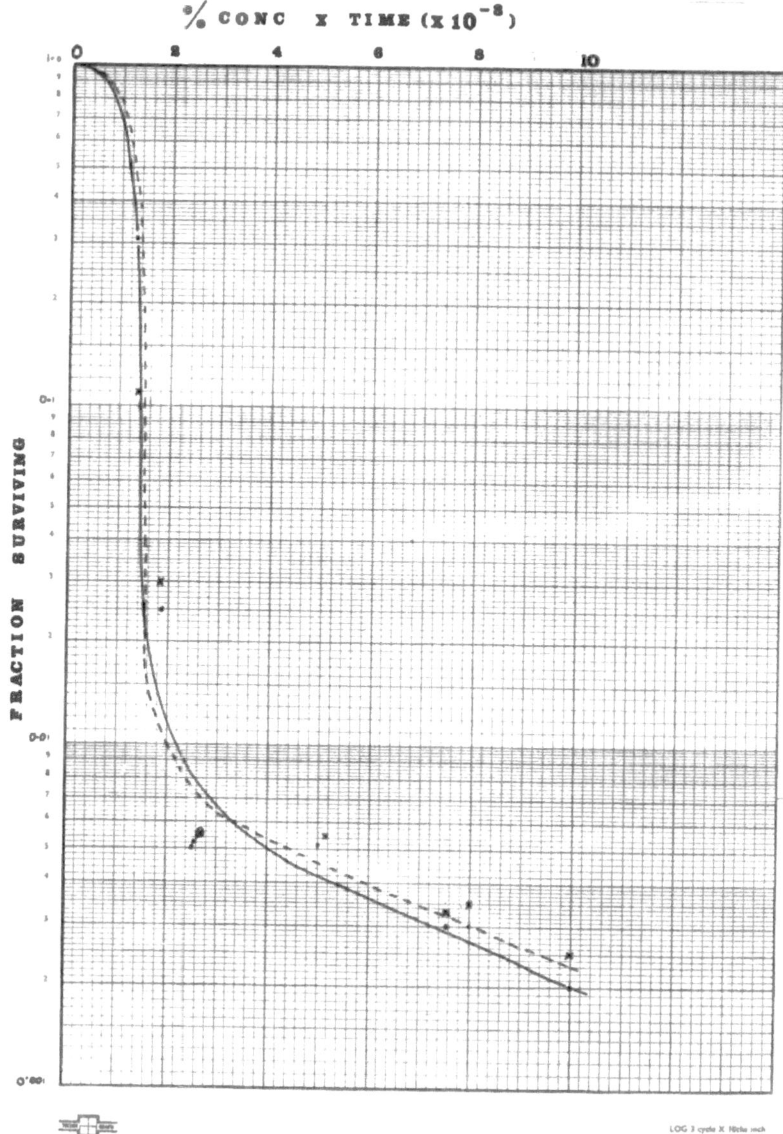

Fig. 8.6: Fraction of cells surviving vincristine
doses of 1 mg/80 ml.(Exp.3).

●----● Model A.
x——x Model B.

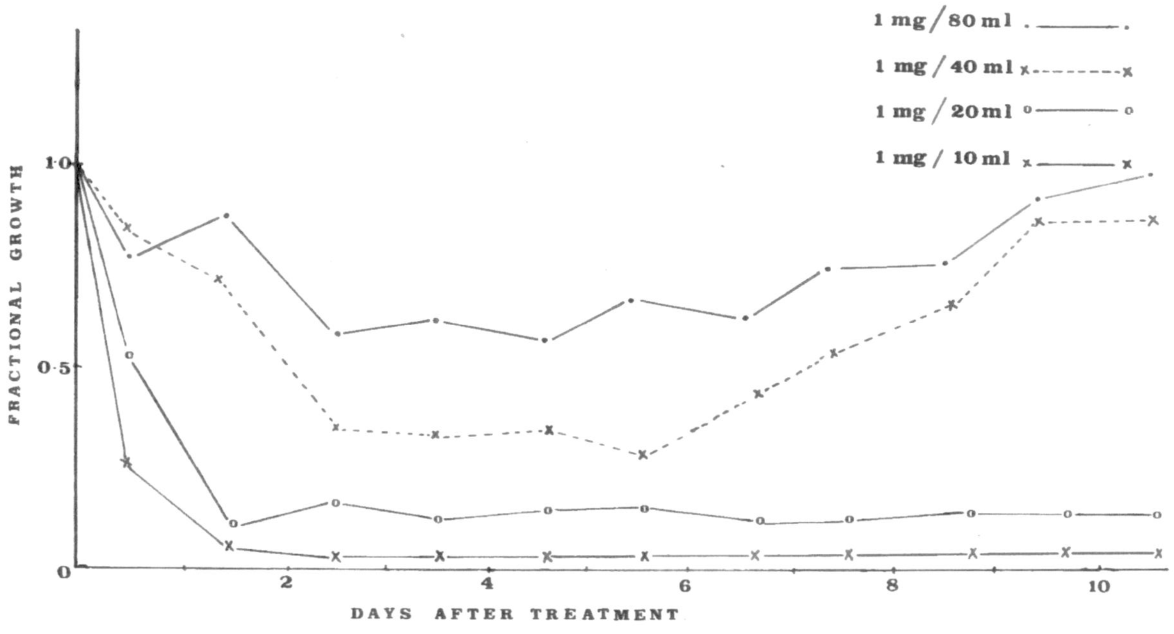

Fig. 8.7: Fractional growth rate of <u>Vicia</u> seedlings after various dosages of vincristine against days after treatment. Various concentrations of the drug were used for a fixed period of time (1 hour) (Exp. 4).

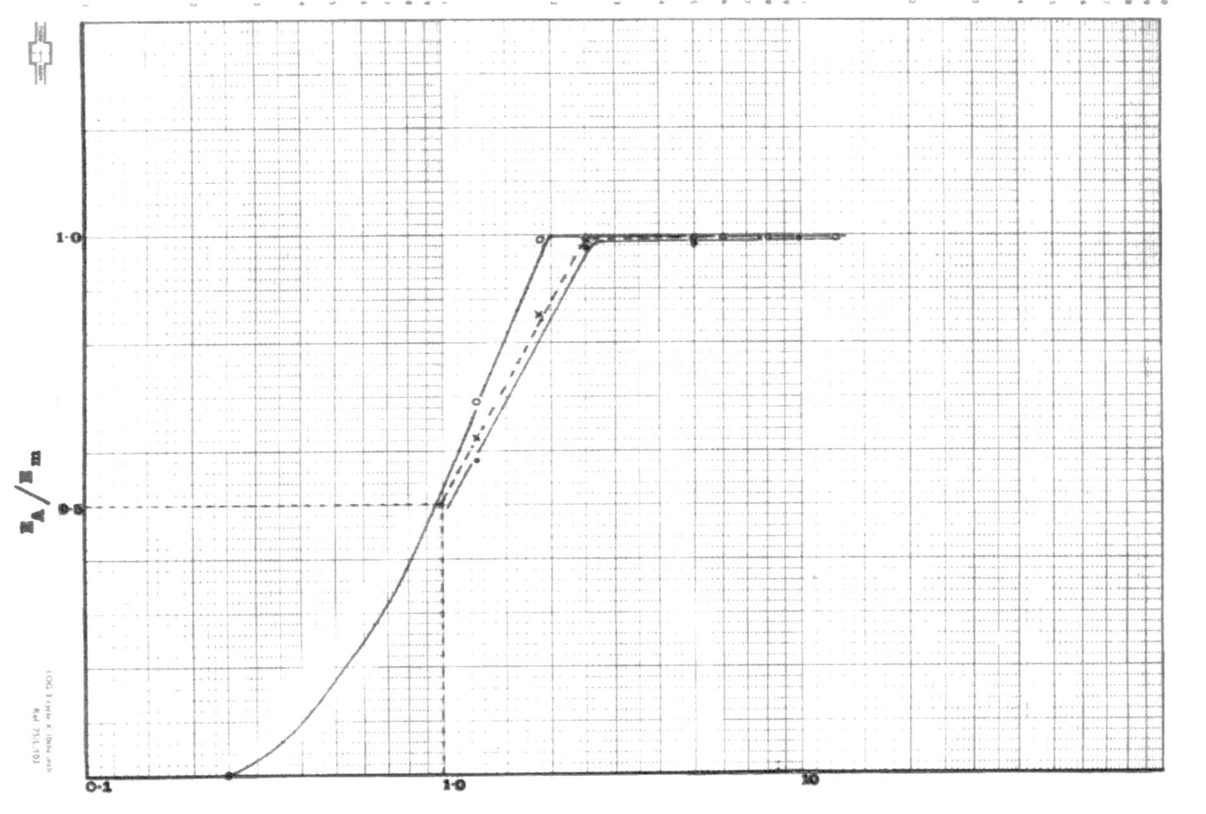

Fig. 8.8 Log-concentration response curves.

    ○————○   1 mg/80 ml (Exp.2)

    x------x   1 mg/40 ml (Exp. 3)

    •————•   One hour exposure to the drug, using different concentrations
                    (Exp. 4). $\dfrac{1}{K_A} = 10^{+3}$

CHAPTER 9.

DISCUSSION

CHAPTER 9.

DISCUSSION.

The Growth Curves.

The growth curves for Vicia exposed to
ionizing radiation in air are shown in Fig. 8.1.
There is an initial decrease in the growth rate
as a fraction of controls of equal age. The
curve then passes through a minimum before
returning to pre-irradiation levels, and in
some cases, even over-shooting. The minimum
value of the growth rate, and the time taken for
recovery depends on the size of the dose.

In order to explain the shape of the growth
curve over the first three days, it is necessary
to take into account the fact that damaged cells
do not die immediately after doses of the order
of a few hundred rads (Puck and Marcus, 1956).
Some succeed in completing two, or even more
divisions, and it is assumed that they are all
capable of differentiating if called upon to do
so. These cells thus make a continuing, though
decreasing contribution to the growth-rate of
the root in the first few days following
irradiation. At the same time the meristematic
cells which retained their reproductive integrity
make an increasing contribution to the growth-rate.
This contribution from the integer cells is

85.

represented by the chained line in Fig. 9.1,
and can be derived from a consideration of
the mathematical models. It is because of
these two processes that the growth-curve has a
minimum value corresponding to the point where
the two contributions are approximately equal,
and are about to interchange their order of
importance.

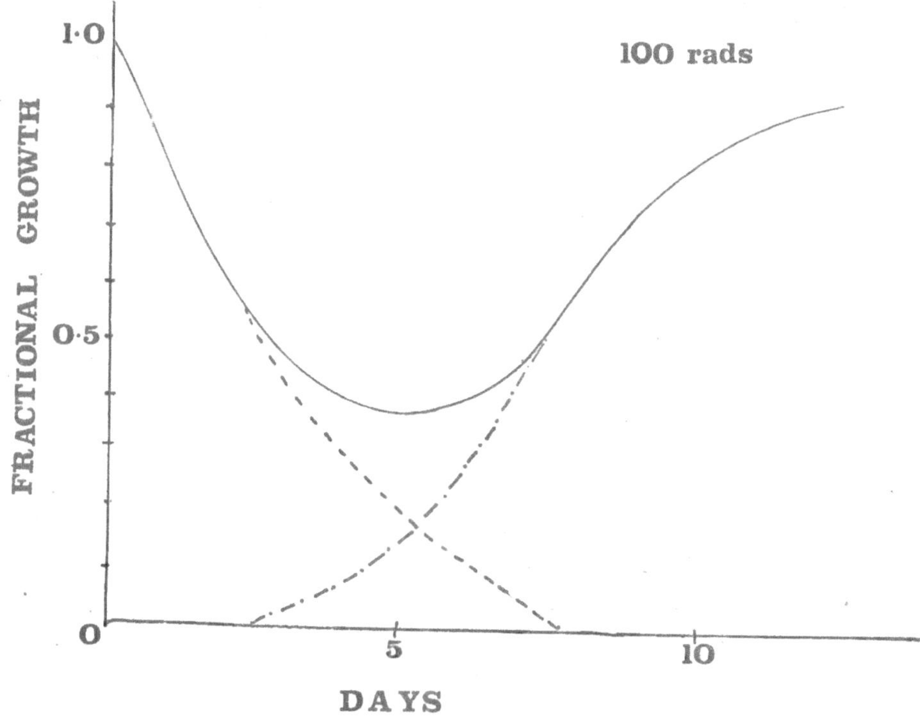

Fig. 9.1. The growth curve of roots exposed
to 100 rads as a fraction of that of controls
(full line) is built up of two components.
The broken line represents the decreasing
contribution of cells which have lost their
reproductive integrity; the chained line
represents the increasing contribution of
integer cells.

<u>Dose response curves with respect to
reproductive integrity</u>.

The dose response curves of the <u>Vicia</u>
seedlings irradiated in air were deduced
as described in Chapter 3 and Appendix B and
C, using Models A and B. The basis for these
models is that, when the number of meristematic
cells is less than normal as a result of
radiation-induced cell death, then the
<u>proportion</u> of cells which differentiate in
a time interval is also less than normal. Thus,
an excess of cells undergoing division is
provided, over those lost by differentiation,
so that repopulation of the meristem can take
place.

The curve obtained when the fraction of
cells surviving radiation dosage is plotted
against the dose, is of the sigmoid or "type C"
form, in that the curve is composed of an initial
pseudothreshold, or shoulder region, followed
by a region of exponential decline. (Fig. 8.2).

The shape of the dose response curve
obtained is similar to one which has been
reported to fit the observed data on the x-ray
dose response curve for reproductive integrity
of mammalian cells (Puck and Marcus, 1956;
Berry, 1969).

The mathematical form of the curve is the following:

$$S = 1 - \left\{ 1 - \exp(-D/D_o) \right\}^m \quad \ldots\ldots\ldots 9.1.$$

and $\ln S = \ln m - D/D_o$ (see Chapter 2)

The intercept, m, on the Y-axis was found to be 1.5 and 1.8 using Models A and B respectively. Here each biological unit presents m targets, and each of these m targets must receive n hits to cause the unit to react. Assuming that only one hit is required in each of m targets, the fraction of cells surviving can be represented by equation 9.1. This equation is of the form corresponding to a multi-target model (each target requiring one hit for inactivation).

The 37 per cent dose slope was found to be 40 rads. This is in agreement with results obtained by Hall (1962), where intercept m was found to be either 3 or 4, with a corresponding dose slope of 40-43 rads. G_{10} and G_{min} values (Table 8.1) are also in close agreement with those obtained by Hall (1962).

<u>The Mode of action of vincristine</u>.

When <u>Vicia</u> seedlings were exposed to a fixed
concentration of vincristine for varying lengths of time,
and also, when, for a fixed period of time seedlings were
exposed to varying concentrations of the drug, growth curve
were obtained. (Figs. 8.4 and 8.7). These curves were
found to be similar to those when <u>Vicia</u> seedlings were
exposed to increasing doses of ionizing radiation. The
growth rates decreased initially, and passed through a
minimum value, before recovering to the pre-treatment
levels. In the cases where the drug doses were too sever
for recovery to take place, (e.g. 1 mg vincristine/40 ml
water for three hours), the growth rate decreased and
remained at a low level without any subsequent recovery.
The same effect was observed when <u>Vicia</u> seedlings were
exposed to doses of ionizing x-irradiation exceeding 200
rads.

As the drug-dose to the bean root was increased, G_{mi}
decreased. This decrease in G_{min} was also observed when
seedlings were exposed to increasing doses of ionizing
radiation.

Because the growth curves following drug administration are similar to those following radiation dosages, one
is justified in using similar parameters in drug studies,
i.e. G_{10} and G_{min}.

Postulates, similar to those of Models A and B which
describe the response of the meristem to radiation, will
therefore also describe the response of the meristem to dr

Following drug administration, the number of meristematic cells would be less than normal as a result of drug-induced cell death. Therefore the proportion of cells which differentiate in a given time is also less than normal. The proportion of cells dividing in a given time-interval is unimpaired, and the meristem gradually becomes re-populated.   As recovery progresses, the compartment approaches its normal size and the rate of differentiation and hence root growth, returns to its steady state values.

Using Models A and B, survival curves, depicting the fraction of cells surviving drug-administration have been derived.   (Figs. 8.5 and 8.6).

The Shape of the Survival Curves.

Sigmoid survival curves were obtained when meristematic Vicia cells were exposed to varying doses of vincristine. The curve is composed of an initial shoulder followed by a region of steep exponential decline.   A second, slower, exponential decrease is observed at higher doses.

The term "fraction surviving" represents that fraction of meristematic Vicia cells which have not combined with the vincristine molecules.   The term "dose" used in the drug studies is a product of the concentration of the dose (in mg/ml) and the time of exposure of the seedlings to the drug. As in drug-receptor theory (Chapter 5) the vincristine molecules are assumed to be in excess, and occupation with receptor molecules does not alter the concentration of the drug.

The survival curves obtained through radiation studies
may be superficially compared with those obtained through
drug studies:-

The initial exponential portion of the drug curves
could be matched with the radiation survival curves. It
should therefore be possible to read off the extrapolation
number of the drug curve and compare it with the extrapolation number obtained from the radiation dose-response
curve.

Straight-line regressions were fitted to the data
of Tables 8.7 and 8.8. In the case of 1 mg/80 ml, the
extrapolation number was found to be 35.6. This correspond
closely to the extrapolation number obtained when 1 mg/40 m
was used for half the periods of time, of 41.4. For radiation, the intercept on the Y-axis was found to be 1.5 and
1.8 using Models A and B respectively. The fact that the
extrapolation number is higher for drugs than it is for
radiation, implies that, in the case of cytotoxic agents
on cells, there are many more "receptor sites" per cell th
in the case of radiation on cells.

The 37% dose slope, i.e. the mean lethal dose for
radiation was found to be 40 rads. In the case of the dru
for a concentration of 1 mg/40 ml, this value was found
to be 4.8 minutes, and for half the drug concentration,
i.e. 1 mg/80 ml, the mean lethal dose was found to be 9
minutes.

The shoulder obtained on the radiation survival curve
is an indication of the sublethal repair that takes place
immediately after cells have been "hit". For drugs, the
magnitude of the width of the shoulder could be an indicat

of the time necessary to penetrate the cells and to inactivate them. Therefore a comparison of the width of the shoulders of the two types of survival curves can not be made, because of the two different mechanisms involved.

The second, slower decrease of the drug-survival curve could possibly be due to the deeply situated cells in the Quiescent Centre. These cells would become inactivated, provided that the time of exposure to the drug is long enough. In the case of radiation on meristematic _Vicia_ cells, it has been shown (Clowes, 1959) that cells in the Q.C. form a "reservoir" of cells which are less vulnerable because of their quiescence, but are able to restart DNA synthesis and division when normal meristematic cells stop. Therefore, it is thought that, as in the case of radiation, cells in the Q.C. probably are relatively insensitive to the action of vincristine due to their situation within the meristem, or due to the fact that they divide more slowly than other meristematic cells.

Another possible explanation for the slower decrease in the survival curve is that a second type of receptor exists which is less sensitive to vincristine. Once these receptors have been saturated by the drug molecules, the subsequent slow decline in survival follows.

<u>Pharmacological Dose-Response Curves</u>:

By using Models A and B, the fraction of cells surviving drug dosages have been calculated.   As in Chapters 5 and 8, let E_m represent the maximum effect of the drug, i.e. total number of cells occupied.

Let E_A represent the "effect" induced by a certain concentration of the drug [A].

Fig. 8.8 depicts the fraction of cells occupied against log vincristine dosage, i.e. E_A/E_m. The dose response-curves thus obtained are similar to those in Fig 5.1 which were deduced from equation 5.5.

On a log-dose scale, S-shaped curves were obtained (Fig. 8.8).   These curves are of similar shape to the theoretical log concentration-response curves.

From the dose-response curves obtained experimentally, the "affinity", $\frac{1}{K_A}$, of the vincristine molecules to the <u>Vicia</u> receptors could be found.   The affinity of a drug to receptors is constant for a specific drug. $\frac{1}{K_A}$ should therefore be independent on the mode of drug-administration.

$\frac{1}{K_A}$ was found to be of constant value in both the experiments in which a constant concentration was used for varying lengths of time, (Experiments 2 and 3) as well as in Experiment 4 where, for a fixed time, different concentrations of the drug was used. From Fig. 8.8, K_A was found to correspond to a vincristine dosage of 1×10^{-3}

The "affinity" of vincristine to the receptors, i.e.

$\frac{1}{K_A}$, is thus $\frac{1}{10^{-3}} = 10^{+3}$.

(The affinity of the drug to the cells is expressed as a fraction without units.) It can be assumed that vincristine acts on meristematic _Vicia_ cells under equilibrium conditions, and therefore equation 5.5 is valid for this system.

Because only one drug was used, the "intrinsic" activity of vincristine relative to another drug could not be obtained.

For comparative purposes, a similar dose-response curve was drawn for radiation-induced cell mutation. (Fig. 8.3).   Here, the dosage corresponding to a response equal to half the maximum response, was found to be 40 rads.   The "affinity" of radiation to vincristine molecules is therefore $\frac{1}{40} (\text{rads})^{-1}$.

Oliver (1962) had found that both Models A and B approximate the true kinetics of the meristem after irradiation.

On the action of drugs on receptors, both Models A and B (which were used to determine the fraction of cells occupied by the vincristine molecules), because they accurately represent the mode of action of drugs on receptors, are therefore reliable models of the cell kinetics pertaining in the meristem.

<u>From Fig. 8.8 the following deductions can be made:-</u>

i) An increase in the drug dose results in an increase of
the quantity of cells inactivated by the drug. This
obeys the pharmacological law, where an increase in the
concentration of the drug results in an increase of the
fraction of drug-receptor complexes. Hence equation 5.5
is obeyed in this respect.

ii) Since the number of specific receptors in the meristem is
limited, the maximum amount of cells that is able to
become inactivated, is limited as well. From Fig. 8.8,
a saturation of the receptors is observed after a certain
drug dosage has been reached. This again obeys the
pharmacological laws laid down in Chapter 5, where, the
maximal amount of drug-receptor complexes is limited. An
increase of the concentration of the drug causes a saturation of the receptors.

iii) Equation 5.5, which gives the relation between the fraction
of cells occupied, and the concentration of the drug, is
valid as long as a gradual increase of the dose of the drug
results in a gradual saturation of the receptor system.
In the experiments on <u>Vicia faba</u>, the time taken for the
cells to be saturated, varied with the different concentrations. For a concentration of 1 mg/80 ml, the saturation
time was about 1 hour (Table 8.8), while for 1 mg/40 ml,
the time for saturation was between 0.5 and 1 hour. (Table
8.7 and Fig. 8.8).
These deductions are further proof that the pharmacologica:
laws were obeyed when Models A and B were used to determine
the fraction of cells surviving vincristine dosages.

<u>Comparison of cell-death induced by drugs with that induced by ionizing radiation:-</u>

i) The drug acts via the occupation of specific receptors. It is assumed that receptor sites are of the same order of magnitude as the drug molecules, whereby, in the simplest case, a reversible bi-molecular reaction occurs between drugs and receptors. In radiation studies, the mode of action is assumed to be irreversible, although sub-lethal recovery occurs immediately after the cells have been exposed to radiation.

ii) For drug studies, each cell is assumed to have a number of receptor sites allied to it. Before a cell is complete-ly inactivated, each receptor site has to be occupied by a drug molecule. It was found that the number of receptor sites per cell is of the order of 45 for vincristine on meristematic <u>Vicia</u> cells.
Similarly, with radiation studies, each cell has $\underline{m}$ targets. Before a cell is sterilised, it must receive at least $\underline{n}$ hits in each of its $\underline{m}$ targets.

iii) One molecule of drug is assumed to react with 1 receptor molecule. Similarly, for radiation, in the multi-target single-hit theory, one hit is required to inactivate one target. ($n = 1$)

iv) It is assumed that all the individual receptors in question have the same "affinity" to the drug molecules, and that occupation of some receptors does not interfere in any way with the chance of interaction with the unoccupied ones.

97.

In radiation theory, the x-rays are very penetrative,
and the same condition holds as with drug theory.

v) The term "dose" for vincristine acting on meristematic
<u>Vicia</u> cells is given as a product of the concentration
of the drug (in mg/ml) and the time that the cells are
exposed to the drug.   "Dose" in radiation theory is given
in terms of rads, i.e. the dosage absorbed by the tissue.
The time that the cells are exposed to radiation is
negligible compared to the time that cells are exposed
to the drug.

SUMMARY

SUMMARY.

Models A and B are two mathematical models which
have been successfully used in the past to find the
fraction of meristematic _Vicia_ cells surviving radiation
dosages.

Vicia seedlings, exposed to varying doses of vincristine, yielded growth curves similar to those obtained when
exposed to ionizing x-irradiation.

Because of the similarity of the growth curves, it
was felt that similar parameters, i.e. G_{10} and G_{min},
and eventually Models A and B, could be used to explain
the response of the meristem to drugs.

Dose-response curves were thus obtained, but these
were different from those obtained through x-irradiation
studies. In both cases, an initial shoulder to the curves
were observed, followed by a region of exponential decline.
In the case of drugs, however, a second, slower, exponen-
tially declining component was observed.

The radiation-and drug-survival curves could be
superficially compared with each other: the extrapolation
number, m (i.e. the number of targets per cell), as well
as the mean lethal dose of the two functions, could be
determined.   For radiation, $m = 1.4$, whereas for the
drug, $m = 35.6$ and $m = 41.4$ (using 1 mg/80 ml and
1 mg/40 ml respectively). The fact that the extrapolation
number is higher for drugs than it is for radiation,
implies that, in the case of cytotoxic agents on cells,
there are many more "receptor sites" per cell than in the

case of radiation on cells. The 37% dose slope
(i.e. the mean lethal dose) for radiation was found to
be 40 rads. For a vincristine dose of 1 mg/40 ml, this
value corresponded to an exposure time of 4.5 minutes,
and for 1 mg/80 ml, the time of exposure of the drug to
the cells was 9 minutes. The magnitude of the width
of the shoulders of the survival curves could not be
compared, because of the different modes of action of
radiation and drugs.

The dose-response curves based on Models A and B
were found to be similar to the curves based on the action
of drugs on receptors. The drug-receptor theory was
adapted specifically to explain the action of vincristine
on _Vicia_ meristematic cells. A value for the "affinity"
of the drug to _Vicia_ cells was deduced according to the
drug-receptor laws. A comparative value for the "affinity"
of radiation to _Vicia_ cells was also deduced. The
"affinity" was found to be 10^{+3} and $\frac{1}{40}$ (rads)$^{-1}$ for
vincristine and radiation respectively.

Analogies were drawn between the theoretical dose-
response curves and those obtained experimentally. These
suggest that the cell-kinetic assumptions made in Models
A and B accurately represent the cell population kinetics
of meristematic _Vicia_ cells, thus substantiating Olivers'
work on radiation.